Wound Healing

Wound Healing

Edited by

HERWIG JANSSEN, RAOUL ROOMAN and J.I.S. ROBERTSON

Janssen Research Foundation, 2340-Beerse, Belgium

WRIGHTSON BIOMEDICAL PUBLISHING LTD

Petersfield

Editorial Office:

Wrightson Biomedical Publishing Ltd
Ash Barn House, Winchester Road, Stroud,
Petersfield, Hampshire GU32 3PN, UK
Telephone: 0730 65647

Distributors:

Blackwell Scientific Publications
Osney Mead, Oxford OX2 0EL, UK
Telephone: 0865 240201

Year Book Medical Publishers
200 North LaSalle Street, Chicago,
Illinois 60601, USA
Telephone: 312 726 9733

British Library Cataloguing in Publication Data

Wound Healing.
  1. Humans. Wounds. Healing
  I. Janssen, Herwig II. Rooman, Raoul III. Robertson, J.
  I. S.
  617.14

  ISBN 1 871816 10 6

Phototypeset by Scribe Design, Gillingham, Kent
Printed in Great Britain by Biddles Ltd, Guildford.

Contents

Pathophysiology of Chronic Wounds

Clinical Wound Healing Research

Summary

Contributors

G. Apodaca, *Department of Anatomy, University of California, San Francisco, CA 94143-0750, USA*

M.J. Banda, *Laboratory of Radiobiology and Environmental Health, LR 102, University of California, San Francisco, CA 94143–0750, USA*

A. Barbul, *Department of Surgery, Sinai Hospital, 2401 W. Belvedere Avenue, Baltimore, MD 21215, USA*

K.N. Broadley, *Department of Pathology, Vanderbilt University School of Medicine, 21st and Garland Avenue, Nashville, TN 37232, USA*

C.G. Caday, *CNS Growth Factor Research Laboratory, Massachusetts General Hospital – East, Boston, MA 02114, USA*

M. Chi, *Laboratory of Developmental Biology and Anomalies, National Institutes of Dental Research, National Institutes of Health, Building 30 Room 414, Bethesda, MD 20892, USA*

R.A.F. Clark, *University of Colorado School of Medicine, Division of Dermatology and Pediatrics, National Jewish Center for Immunology and Respiratory Medicine, Denver, CO 80206, USA*

F. Croute, *Dermatology Clinic and Inserm U.209, E. Herriot Hospital, F69374 Lyon Cedex 03, France*

J.M. Davidson, *Department of Pathology, Vanderbilt University School of Medicine, 21st and Garland Avenue, Nashville, TN 37232, USA*

E. Delaporte, *Dermatology Clinic and Inserm U.209, E. Herriot Hospital, F69374 Lyon Cedex 03, France*

B. Fagrell, *Karolinska Institute, Department of Medicine, Danderyd Hospital, S-182 88 Danderyd, Sweden*

S.P. Finklestein, *CNS Growth Factor Research Laboratory, Massachusetts General Hospital – East, Boston, MA 02114, USA*

G. Gabbiani, *Department of Pathology, University of Geneva, CMU, 1 rue Michel Servet, 1211 Geneva 4, Switzerland*

M. Gaucherand, *Dermatology Clinic and Inserm U.209, E. Herriot Hospital, F69374 Lyon Cedex 03, France*

A.W. Goode, *Surgical Unit, The London Hospital, Whitechapel, London E1 1BB, UK*

W.H. Goodson III, *Department of Surgery, University of California, San Francisco, CA 94143–0522, USA*

F. Gottrup, *Department of Surgical Gastroenterology K, Odense University Hospital, DK-5000 Odense C, Denmark*

D. Hartman, *Radioanalysis Centre, Pasteur Institute, Lyon, France*

M. Heckmann, *Dermatology Clinic, Ludwig Maximilians University, Frauenlobstrasse 9–11, 8000 Munich 2, Germany*

G.S. Herron, *Department of Dermatology, University of California, San Francisco, CA 94143-0750, USA*

E.W. Howard, *Laboratory of Radiobiology and Environmental Health, LR 102, University of California, San Francisco, CA 94143–0750, USA*

T.K. Hunt, *Department of Surgery, University of California, 513 Parnassus, HSE Room 839, San Francisco, CA 94143–0522, USA*

M. Klagsbrun, *Departments of Surgery and Biological Chemistry, Children's Hospital Medical Center, 320 Longwood Avenue, Boston, MA 02115, USA*

Th. Krieg, *Dermatology Clinic, Ludwig Maximilians University, Frauenlobstrasse 9–11, 8000 Munich 2, Germany*

M. Kulozik, *Dermatology Clinic, Ludwig Maximilians University, Frauenlobstrasse 9–11, 8000 Munich 2, Germany*

Ch. M. Lapière, *Department of Dermatology, CHU Sart Tilman, University of Liège, B-4000, Liège, Belgium*

G.R. Martin, *National Institutes on Aging, Gerontology Research Center, 4945 Eastern Avenue, Baltimore, MD 21224, USA*

C. Mauch, *Dermatology Clinic, Ludwig Maximilians University, Frauenlobstrasse 9–11, 8000 Munich 2, Germany*

G. Murphy, *Strangeways Research Laboratory, Cambridge CB1 4RN, UK*

J.F. Nicolas, *Dermatology Clinic and Inserm U.209, E. Herriot Hospital, F69374 Lyon Cedex 03, France*

J. Niinikoski, *Department of Surgery, University of Turku, SF-20520 Turku 52, Finland*

E.J. O'Keefe, *Department of Dermatology, University of North Carolina, USA*

G.F. Pierce, *Department of Experimental Pathology, Amgen Inc., Thousand Oaks, CA, USA*

J. Pouysségur, *Biochemical Research Centre, CNRS – UPR 7300, University of Nice-Sophia Antipolis, Parc Valrose, 06034 Nice Cedex, France*

M.C. Regan, *Department of Surgery, Johns Hopkins Medical Institute, Baltimore, MD, USA*

R. Reich, *Laboratory of Developmental Biology and Anomalies, National Institutes of Dental Research, National Institutes of Health, Building 30 Room 414, Bethesda, MD 20892, USA*

M. Richard, *Biochemistry Laboratory B, E. Herriot Hospital, F69374 Lyon Cedex 03, France*

J.I.S. Robertson, *Department of Medicine, Prince of Wales Hospital, Chinese University of Hong Kong, and Janssen Research Foundation, B-2340 Beerse, Belgium*

R. Rudolph, *Division of Plastic and Reconstructive Surgery, Scripps Clinic and Research Foundation, La Jolla, CA 92037–1093, USA*

T.J. Ryan, *Department of Dermatology, The Slade Hospital, Headington, Oxford OX3 7JH, UK*

A.C. Sank, *Laboratory of Developmental Biology and Anomalies, National Institutes of Dental Research, National Institutes of Health, Building 30 Room 414, Bethesda, MD 20892, USA*

Y. Sarret, *Department of Dermatology, Stanford University Medical Center, R 144, Stanford, CA 94305, USA*

K. Scharffetter, *Dermatology Clinic, Ludwig Maximilians University, Frauenlobstrasse 9–11, 8000 Munich 2, Germany*

H. Scheuenstuhl, *Department of Surgery, University of California, San Francisco, CA 94143–0522, USA*

K. Seuwen, *Biochemical Research Centre, CNRS – UPR 7300, University of Nice-Sophia Antipolis, Parc Valrose, 06034 Nice Cedex, France*

T. Shima, *Laboratory of Developmental Biology and Anomalies, National Institutes of Dental Research, National Institutes of Health, Building 30 Room 414, Bethesda, MD 20892, USA*

J. Thivolet, *Dermatology Clinic and Inserm U.209, E. Herriot Hospital, F69374 Lyon Cedex 03, France*

J.E. Tooke, *Post Graduate Medical Centre, Royal Devon and Exeter Hospital, Exeter EX2 5DW, UK*

J. Vande Berg, *Core Electron Microscopy Laboratory, Veterans Administration Medical Center, La Jolla, CA 92037-1093, USA*

M.S. Walsh, *Surgical Unit, The London Hospital, Whitechapel, London E1 1BB, UK*

D.T. Woodley, *Department of Dermatology, Stanford University Medical Center, R 144, Stanford, CA 94305, USA*

Preface

In just a few years, enormous progress has been made in our understanding of the molecular and cellular processes involved in tissue repair. Molecular biological techniques have greatly simplified the characterization of a variety of growth factors, enzymes and structural proteins thought to be important in wound healing. New cell culture techniques have made it possible to study each cellular component separately and to investigate their interactions. Sufficiently large amounts of growth factors and structural proteins are now produced by the biotechnological industry to start animal experiments and limited clinical trials. The resultant expansion of our knowledge on wound healing and the availability of new treatment modalities have renewed the interest of clinicians in the problems of chronic skin ulcers.

On 2–4 November 1989, a group of experts from Europe and the USA gathered in the old priory of Corsendonk (Belgium) to discuss recent progress in wound healing. The group included both fundamental scientists and physicians and the discussion ranged from nucleotide sequences of genes to the method of choice for measuring wound size in clinical trials.

This volume contains an account of the papers presented at that meeting. The book has been organized in four sections. The first gives a brief overview of the processes involved in tissue repair. The next section is devoted to the molecular and cellular biology of wound healing and deals with the regulation of granulation tissue formation, keratinocyte migration, myofibroblast biology and wound contraction. The pathophysiology of chronic wounds and the importance of an adequate oxygen supply are discussed in the third section. The final part takes up wound healing research in man and the important question of measurement of wound size.

The book attempts to bridge the gap between cell biologists and clinicians and should therefore be of interest to both scientists and physicians who care for patients with chronic skin ulcers. We hope that this publication will help the reader to keep up with this most important, and rapidly progressing field.

We are grateful to the contributors, not only for their papers, which are published here, but also for their lucidity and discipline in verbal presentation at the meeting; to the chairmen of the various sessions for their stimulus and authority; to Janssen and Ethicon companies for financial support; to the Janssen Research Council, under whose aegis the symposium was convened; and finally to Dr Paul Janssen for his continued interest and encouragement.

THE EDITORS

Overview of Wound Repair

Wound Healing
Edited by H. Janssen, R. Rooman and J.I.S. Robertson
© 1991 Wrightson Biomedical Publishing Ltd

1

Genetics and Tissue Repair

CH. M. LAPIÈRE

Department of Dermatology, CHU Sart Tilman, University of Liège, Belgium

Healing is the reaction of any multicellular organism, allowing the preservation of the boundary between its inner content and the extracellular environment, maintaining the integrity of the organs required for locomotion and ensuring the continuity of the support of the parenchymal, endothelial and epithelial cells. Healing is required for survival in an ever aggressive environment.

HEALING IS INDUCED BY SEVERAL MECHANISMS

Several types of conditions that modify the homeostatic equilibrium of cells will trigger the healing reaction. They are characterized by the loss of communication between the cells, or between cells and their support, or by cell death.

Epithelial or parenchymal cells exchange information among themselves as well as with mesenchymal cells through gap junctions or by the release of cytokines. Any alterations of this biological information caused by loss of cell–cell contact or by dilution of mediators are potential triggers of a cellular reaction.

Disruption of the lateral association of the bundles of collagen polymers without alteration of blood vessels or epithelial cells as observed in striae distensae will never lead to the formation of a scar. A trauma produced by a sharp instrument induces minimal cell death and, when the edges of the wound are well fastened, the loss of continuity is minor. The healing reaction will however occur, with little inflammation and angiogenesis, by a persistent activation of the connective tissue cells sometimes quite far from the section. The mechanism consists in a remodeling of the fibrous network that ultimately allows bridging of the two sides of the wound (see Chapter 4). The difference between the two conditions might be in part related to changes in the mechanical information that mesenchymal cells receive from their support (Lapière and Nusgens, 1989), undisturbed in the former and modified in the latter. Mechanical sensing is a known process significant in the behaviour of several types of cells (see Chapter 14).

Removal of the superficial layer of skin as in split thickness wounds as opposed to full thickness wounds induces healing with a minimum formation of granulation tissue. The rate of covering by the epithelial cells, rapid in the former and delayed in the latter, might make the difference. Epithelial–mesenchymal interaction might represent the mechanism controlling the extent of granulation tissue formation. Epithelial cytokines modulate the functions of fibroblasts (see Chapter 8).

Most often a loss of continuity is accompanied by extravasation of blood cells in the connective tissue. Blood clotting and the release of cytokines and breakdown products from the clot will lead to a complex reaction and the formation of granulation tissue maturing into a scar. A similar reaction can be triggered by a large variety of stimuli such as toxic agents, bacteria or viruses, immune mediated reactions, or death of any type of cell in any location of the organism. The common denominator of all these pathogenic agents is cell death and the release of cytokines. The healing reaction terminates when physiological equilibrium is recovered. It should therefore be considered as a homeostatic mechanism.

HEALING IN HERITABLE DISEASES

There is a large array of heritable connective tissue disorders that affect the mechanical properties of supporting structures in man and animals. Skin, bone, tendon, blood vessels, ocular membranes and gingiva can all be altered. Some of these disorders are defined up to the molecular level and related to defective connective tissue macromolecules. Although wounds, ruptures or fractures can be fatal in these disorders, the healing reaction can always potentially occur and lead to the formation of a scar. Dermatosparaxis in animals (Hanset and Lapière, 1974) such as the calf or the sheep, is an example of a heritable condition in which fragility of skin is so extensive that minor trauma induces large wounds, necrosis and infection which result in death. When mechanical protection is offered to the animal smaller wounds will heal and life can be preserved.

There exists in man or animals no heritable disorder characterized by an absence of healing. Some diseases, whose numbers are few, are characterized by impaired healing such as the congenital deficiency in factor XIII in which healing occurs but the scar is very fragile. Some acquired disorders such as scurvy, in which a deficient formation of collagen depends upon a lack of activity of enzymes requiring ascorbic acid as a cofactor, result in delayed healing and fragile scars. The absence of congenital healing defects supports the concept that the mechanisms involved in the process of healing are so fundamental that their significant impairment could not permit survival.

THE REDUNDANT MECHANISMS AND CONTROLS IN TISSUE REPAIR

The basic cellular mechanisms required for healing are similar to those involved in development, growth and ageing. They are chemokinesis, cell multiplication and differentiation. These processes and their controls can be observed in a time sequence analysis of the healing of a full thickness skin wound.

Within seconds after wounding, there is formation of a blood clot. Its impairment does not represent a limiting factor in the process since it is known that patients defective in certain coagulation factors, for example haemophiliacs, will heal, but slowly.

Within hours there is a migration of cells from the surrounding blood vessels to the clot. Chemokinesis depends on a large number of variables involving the extracellular matrix, chemical mediators and the locomotor apparatus of the cell. Messages pass through membrane receptors (see Chapter 2) and sensors of gradient of bioactive molecules, a mechanism that is of prime importance in development and organogenesis. The absence of one of them or a defect in its recognition at the membrane level would probably not seriously impair the overall reaction.

In a matter of days, endothelial and mesenchymal cells attracted to the clot will multiply and form the granulation tissue composed of new blood vessels and supporting connective tissue. The mechanisms involved in cell multiplication and control are obviously of prime importance in the development and growth of a multicellular organism. The multiplicity of the mediators acting through membrane receptors (see Chapter 5) on the cell machinery and involved in cell division is so redundant that the lack of one of them would be insufficient to suppress the reaction.

In a matter of weeks, contraction of the wound occurs and is related to the activity of the myofibroblasts (see Chapter 11) under the control of various growth factors (see Chapter 12). Even if their contractile activity was missing the healing process would be delayed but not suppressed completely.

The connective tissue and its potential for repair are required mainly to provide the epidermis with a correct support. In a skin wound, as soon as the granulation tissue is formed, a layer of epithelial cells that surround the wound bed will spread on its surface and cells will later start multiplying to reconstruct a functional epidermis upon maturation. The two mechanisms seem to be independent (see Chapter 10) and are required during skin organogenesis.

Each type of cell that participates in the healing reaction can be assigned a defined function. Some of the cells can be deleted since their function can be performed by other types of cells. For example, the secretion of lytic enzymes by endothelial cells (see Chapter 7) can be supplemented by the activity of macrophages. T lymphocytes modulate the formation of the granulation tissue and regulate the final quality of the scar (see Chapter 3). Healing is impaired in their absence but not suppressed. The mechanisms that ensure the function of the cells and their control are also redundant. Among the growth factors present in the wound fluid are several which trigger a similar function on the specific target cells. The signalling mechanism is also very well protected by a large array of membrane receptors operating through different pathways in the control of cell functions (see Chapter 6).

The duplication in the systems operating the control of the main repair and development functions explains why the likelihood of finding a mutation that would allow the development of a multicellular organism and be responsible for a lack of healing reaction is negligible.

ULCERS ARE WOUNDS THAT FAIL TO HEAL

The above mentioned considerations apply to wounds that could be called physiological. In various clinical conditions, the organ that is the object of a trauma can suffer a defect. Under such conditions, the formation of the granulation tissue and the subsequent reconstruction of a stabilized organ will be delayed or suppressed. Examples of such chronic wounds are skin ulcers. In human clinical conditions they are often the result of impaired metabolism (Chapter 15) and especially impaired oxygen supply (Chapters 16 and 17) caused by defective arterial, venous or lymphatic circulation. Such conditions can be reproduced in the experimental animal (see Chapter 13) to produce models useful for pharmacological investigations. A defective vascular supply can be studied at the tip of skin flaps, while impaired metabolism can be produced by corticosteroid or X-irradiation, by scurvy, by diabetes induced by alloxane intoxication, and by decreased cell multiplication caused by cytotoxic drugs. Such models are required for investigating drugs potentially active in promoting wound healing. In the absence of the additional defects that they produce, healing will proceed at an optimal rate that would not allow the demonstration of the efficiency of potentially active compounds.

Ulcers represent a major challenge for medicine (see Chapter 18). A large amount of knowledge is available concerning their pathophysiology and this will permit us to develop new strategies for therapy (see Chapter 19).

2

Cutaneous Wound Repair: A Review with Emphasis on Integrin Receptor Expression

RICHARD A.F. CLARK

University of Colorado School of Medicine, Division of Dermatology and Pediatrics, National Jewish Center for Immunology and Respiratory Medicine, Denver, Colorado, USA

Tissue repair is a requisite sequel of cutaneous injury for the re-establishment of skin homeostasis. In this review I will discuss briefly the events of cutaneous wound repair including some of our recent findings on integrin extracellular matrix (ECM) receptor expression in wound fibroblasts and migrating epidermis. A more comprehensive review of cutaneous wound repair has been published recently (Clark, 1990a).

Severe cutaneous injury causes cell death and blood vessel disruption. Blood extravasation into the skin initiates platelet activation (Terkeltaub and Ginsberg, 1988), and blood coagulation (Furie and Furie, 1988). Platelets facilitate wound repair by promoting haemostasis, blood vessel constriction, and new tissue formation (Table 1). Platelets induce haemostasis through self-aggregation, induction of blood coagulation, and their adherence to blood vessel wall and interstitial ECM. In addition, platelets release biologically active materials. These include the ECM molecules, fibronectin, fibrinogen, thrombospondin, and von Willebrand factor, which are necessary for platelet aggregation and binding to tissue structure (Ginsberg *et al.*,1988); the growth factors, platelet-derived growth factor (PDGF) (Ross *et al.*, 1986),

Table 1. Platelets in wound repair.

Activity	Effect
Aggregation and clot initiation	Haemostasis
Vasoactive mediator release	Blood vessel constriction
Growth factor release	New tissue formation

transforming growth factor-α (TGF-α) (Derynck, 1988), and TGF-β (Sporn *et al.*, 1987), which are necessary for new tissue generation (Table 2); and the vasoactive substances, serotonin, adenosine diphosphate (ADP), calcium, and thromboxin which are necessary for blood vessel constriction to prevent haemorrhage.

Blood coagulation promotes normal wound repair by effecting haemostasis and generating biologically active mediators (Table 3). Mediators generated by coagulation include kallikrein, thrombin, plasmin, fibrinopeptides, fibrin-split products, bradykinin, and the anaphylatoxins C3a and C5a through spill-over activation of the complement cascade. Most of these factors act as chemoattractants to circulating leukocytes bringing them to the site of injury. Thrombin and plasmin are also growth factors for parenchymal cells (Carney and Cunningham, 1978). Dead and dying cells release a variety of substances that may be important for wound repair, such as tissue factor, lactic acid, lactate dehydrogenase, calcium, lysosomal enzymes, and fibroblast growth factor (FGF) (Folkman and Klagsbrun, 1987). Thus, the substances from platelets, blood coagulation and injured cells not only promote vasoregulation, blood clotting and tissue degradation, but also stimulate processes important for new tissue formation such as cell migration and proliferation, and neomatrix formation.

Blood vessels have many diverse roles in wound repair. Not only does the microvascular system bring oxygen and nutrients to the injured tissue so that

Table 2. Growth factors in wound repair.

Growth factor	Effect
Transforming growth factor-α (TGF-α)	Re-epithelialization
Platelet-derived growth factor (PDGF)	Fibroblast chemotaxis, proliferation and contraction
Fibroblast growth factor (FGF)	Fibroblast and epidermal cell proliferation, Angiogenesis
Transforming growth factor-β (TGF-β)	Fibroblast chemotaxis Extracellular matrix production Protease inhibitor production

Table 3. Blood coagulation in wound repair.

Activity	Effect
Fibrin clot formation	Haemostasis
Mediator generation	Leukocyte chemotaxis Cell Proliferation

it might heal, but it also limits blood coagulation and platelet thrombi, initiates clot lysis, facilitates leukocyte diapedesis, and regenerates through a complex series of events called angiogenesis (Table 4).

Several intrinsic activities of intact blood vessel endothelium (Chien, 1989) limit the extent of platelet aggregation and blood coagulation to the wounded area. These include production of prostacyclin, which inhibits platelet aggregation; cell surface inactivation of thrombin; cell surface activation of protein C, an enzyme that degrades coagulation factors V and VIII; and generation of plasminogen activator which initiates clot lysis.

Activated endothelium expresses specific intercellular adhesion molecules on its surface (Tonnesen, 1989; Johnston *et al.*, 1989). These endothelial cell receptors recognize the $\beta2$ integrin family of receptors (MAC-1, LFA-1, and p150) which are 'upregulated' on circulating leukocytes by chemotactic factors emanating from the wound site (Table 5). The interactions of these

Table 4. Endothelial cells in wound repair.

Activity	Effect
Nonthrombogenic surface	Limits coagulation
Prostacyclin release	Limits platelet thrombi
Plasminogen activator release	Clot lysis
Surface expression of cell adhesion molecules	Leukocyte diapedesis
Collagenase release	Basement membrane degradation
Growth factor production	Autocrine stimulation
Migration and proliferation	Angiogenesis
Inherent capacity to form tubes	Blood flow
Extracellular matrix production	Provisional matrix and basement membrane formation

Table 5. The integrin superfamily of receptors.

Nomenclature	Subunits	Receptor function
VLA-1	$\alpha1\beta1$	Laminin binding
VLA-2,GPIaIIa	$\alpha2\beta1$	Collagen binding
VLA-3	$\alpha3\beta1$	Generic ECM binding
VLA-4	$\alpha4\beta1$	Lymphocyte homing
VLA-5	$\alpha5\beta1$	Fibronectin binding
VLA-6	$\alpha6\beta1$	Laminin binding
LFA-1	$\alpha_L\beta2$	Leukocyte–cell adhesion
Mac-1	$\alpha_M\beta2$	Leukocyte–cell adhesion
p150,95	$\alpha_X\beta2$	Leukocyte–cell adhesion
GPIIbIIIa	$\alpha_p\beta3$	Platelet binding to ECM
Vitronectin receptor	$\alpha_v\beta3$	Vitronectin binding

cell–cell receptors are responsible for leukocyte margination at the site of injury.

Within the first few hours neutrophils and monocytes begin to infiltrate the wound. These blood leukocytes are attracted to injured tissue by a variety of chemotactic factors. The major function of neutrophils is to rid the tissue of contaminating bacteria (Table 6). In doing so they often release lysosomal enzymes and other toxic substances that cause additional tissue destruction. When monocytes invade the wound site, they quickly undergo a phenotypic metamorphosis to macrophages (Riches, 1988). Macrophages phagocytose and kill pathogenic organisms and scavenge tissue debris including effete neutrophils (Table 7). They also generate chemotactic factors which recruit additional inflammatory cells and release enzymes which augment tissue degradation. In addition, macrophages can synthesize and secrete factors which are probably critical for new tissue formation such as PDGF, TGF-α, and TGF-β (Madtes *et al.*, 1988). Macrophages can continually produce growth factors as well as debride tissue and, therefore, can promote the transition from inflammation to new tissue formation.

New tissue in a cutaneous wound consists of a neoepidermis and underlying granulation tissue. Granulation tissue formation begins after a lag period of several days and is comprised of macrophages, fibroblasts, neomatrix, and neovasculature. Granulation tissue provides support for the neoepidermis and is the origin of a neodermis.

Fibroblasts produce and organize the major ECM components of the neodermis (Table 8). TGF-β, PDGF, and fragments of matrix proteins such as fibronectin and collagen promote fibroblast migration, while FGF and PDFG stimulate fibroblast proliferation (Clark, 1990a). Once fibroblasts have migrated into the wound, they produce and deposit exuberant quantities

Table 6.   Neutrophils in wound repair.

Activity	Effect
Phagocytosis and killing of micro-organisms	Wound decontamination
Extracellular release of proteases	Tissue destruction

Table 7.   Macrophages in wound repair.

Activity	Effect
Phagocytosis and killing of micro-organisms	Wound decontamination
Phagocytosis of tissue debris	Wound debridement
Growth factor release	New tissue formation

Table 8. Fibroblasts in wound repair.

Activity	Effect
Migration and proliferation	Fibroplasia
ECM production	Connective tissue formation
Growth factor production	Autocrine stimulation
Dynamic linkage between actin bundles and ECM	Tissue contraction
Protease release	ECM remodelling

of fibronectin, types I and III collagen, and hyaluronate. TGF-β is currently believed to be the most important stimulus of fibroblast ECM production (Sporn *et al.*, 1987) and in fact TGF-β appears in wound fibroblasts synchronously with fibronectin matrix assembly and type I procollagen expression (Welch *et al.*, 1990).

In tissue culture TGF-β also induces fibroblast surface membrane expression of fibronectin receptors (Heino *et al.*, 1989) which are in the β_1 integrin family of ECM receptors (Table 5) (Ruoslahti, 1988). All integrin receptors are composed of one α-subunit (molecular weight range from 142 kDa to 180 kDa) and one β-subunit (molecular weight range from 95 kDa to 130 kDa). The α- and β-subunits are always assembled in the plasma membrane as noncovalently bound heterodimers and both subunits have a rather large extracellular domain and a short cytoplasmic domain. The integrin receptors are categorized into three distinct families according to the specific β-subunits present in the heterodimer.

Fibronectin receptors, but not integrin collagen receptors, appear on wound fibroblasts shortly after TGF-β has appeared and fibronectin assembly has begun (Fig. 1). At this time fibroblasts are becoming aligned in a parallel array across the radial axis of the wound and ultrastructural links between fibroblasts and the ECM have become apparent (Fig. 2). Presumably fibronectin receptors are used to 'grasp' the ECM and are a critical part of the ultrastructural links (Welch *et al.*, 1990). Wound fibroblasts at this stage develop thick actin cables along their longitudinal axes. The actin cables presumably generate tension that is transmitted across the wound through the cell–cell and cell–matrix links, causing tissue contraction. By extrapolation from *in vitro* experiments, PDGF and perhaps TGF-β may stimulate the actin-rich fibroblasts to contract the wound (Clark *et al.*, 1989).

Fibroblasts produce a variety of growth factors similar to macrophages (Shipley *et al.*, 1989); thus, once activated appropriately, fibroblasts may be able to sustain their own growth and/or ECM production. This possibility may have great import in fibrocontractive diseases such as scleroderma, cirrhosis, and pulmonary fibrosis. Collagen matrix appears to have a marked negative

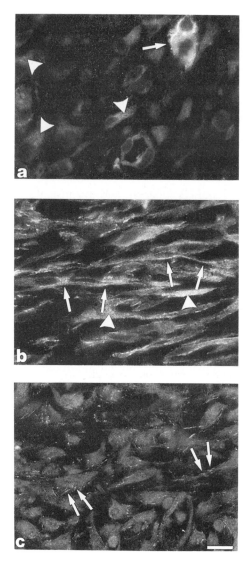

Figure 1. Wound fibroblasts stained with fluorescein-complexed anti-integrin α5β1 antibodies (a and b) and anti-α5 subunit antibodies (c). Photomicrographs were taken of mid-granulation tissue in day 5 (a) and day 7 (b and c) wounds. (a) In day 5 wounds a few fibroblasts stained in a weak perinuclear granular pattern (arrowheads) despite bright peripheral staining of pericytes that surrounded some capillaries (arrow). (b) Striking bright perinuclear granules (arrowheads) and peripheral, linear stitches (arrows) were observed in 7 day wound fibroblasts. (c) Similar peripheral stitch-work staining (arrows), but no perinuclear granular staining, was seen in 7 day wound fibroblasts with antibodies specific for the integrin α5 subunit. Bars, 10 μm.
(Reproduced with permission, from Welch *et al.*, 1990.)

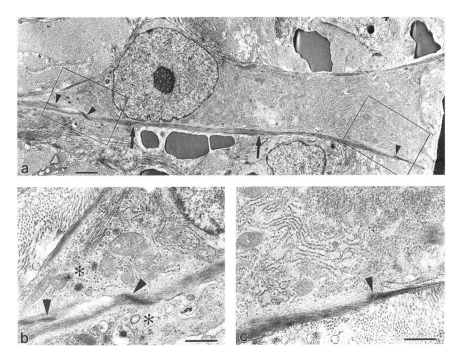

Figure 2. Transmission electron micrograph of a fibroblast in the mid-granulation tissue of a 7 day porcine cutaneous wound. (a) The fibroblast contains a well-organized microfilament bundle (arrows) coursing along the cytoplasmic face of the plasma membrane. The bundle is engaged in cell–cell (enlarged in b) and cell–matrix (enlarged in c) linkages (arrowheads). The left and right rectangles denote the enlarged areas shown in (b) and (c), respectively. (b) Adjacent fibroblasts (asterisks) are linked by a cell–cell adhesion (arrowheads) characterized by 10–20 nm intercellular spacing and 60–75 nm thick cytoplasmic adhesion plaques. (c) The intracellular microfilaments appear to be coaligned with extracellular microfilaments to form a fibronexus (arrowhead). Bars 2μm in (a); 1μm in (b) and (c). (Reproduced with permission, from Welch *et al.*, 1990.)

feedback on collagen production by normal cultured fibroblasts (Mauch *et al.*, 1988), and some evidence exists that this may be true also for cutaneous wound fibroblasts.

New blood vessels form (angiogenesis) concomitantly with ingrowth of fibroblasts and neomatrix deposition (fibroplasia). Morphologically a defined series of events occurs which results in angiogenesis (Ausprunk and Folkman, 1977). Endothelial cells lining the microvasculature adjacent to a wound dissolve the intervening basement membrane and emigrate through the disrupted matrix. Endothelial cells migrate into the newly forming granulation tissue as a cord of cells surrounded by a specialized provisional matrix (Ausprunk *et al.*, 1981; Clark *et al.*, 1982a). Adjacent endothelial cell cords join together forming arcades of new capillaries. Lumina appear within the centre of the arched cords and blood flow begins. Basement membrane rapidly forms between the capillary endothelial cells and granulation tissue neomatrix and thereby replaces the specialized provisional matrix from the wound margin inward toward the tips of capillary sprouts. FGF is partly responsible for angiogenesis through initiating a cascade of events (Mignatti *et al.*, 1989). FGF stimulates endothelial cells to secrete procollagenase and plasminogen activator (PA). The latter enzymatically converts extravasated blood plasminogen to plasmin. Plasmin as well as PA activates procollagenase to collagenase. Together these enzymes can digest the blood vessel basement membrane. Endothelial chemoattractants, such as fibronectin fragments generated from ECM degradation and heparin released from mast cells (Azizkhan *et al.*, 1980), draw endothelial cells through the disrupted basement membrane to form a nascent capillary bud.

Re-epithelialization starts within hours after epidermal disruption, thereby re-establishing the cutaneous barrier to the outside world (Table 9). Epidermal cells from the wound margin and residual hair follicles migrate over the wound surface (Winter, 1962). This lateral motility of epidermal cells across the wound surface is dependent upon an alteration of epidermal cell phenotype including retraction of intracellular keratin filaments, dissolution of intercellular desmosomes (structures that normally interlink epidermal cells confering tensile strength upon the normal epidermis), and formation of peripheral cytoplasmic actin filaments to provide a motor apparatus (Gabbiani *et al.*, 1978). Migrating epidermal cells transit over a provisional matrix containing fibrin and fibronectin (Clark *et al.*, 1982b) while expressing fibronectin receptors (Table 5) (Clark, 1990b). Epidermal cells have the capacity to deposit fibronectin in the extracellular matrix *in vivo* (Grimwood *et al.*, 1988). TGF-β may stimulate the migrating epidermal cells to produce fibronectin (Wikner *et al.*, 1988) and fibronectin receptors and as well as other integrin ECM receptors (Heino *et al.*, 1989; Ignotz *et al.*, 1989), and thereby promote translocation (Nickoloff *et al.*, 1988) over the surface of the wound.

Table 9. Epidermal cells in wound repair.

Activity	Effect
Migration and proliferation	Re-epithelialization
Protease release	Dissection under clot and nonviable tissue
ECM production	Provisional matrix and basement membrane formation
Growth factor production	Autocrine stimulation

Within a day or two after injury, epidermal cells at the wound margin begin to proliferate, providing the migrating epidermis with a new supply of cells. Epidermal growth factor (EGF) or TGF-α is likely to provide the signal for this proliferation (Cohen, 1965; Barrandon and Green, 1987). As re-epithelialization is established, a new basement membrane forms from the wound margin inward, binding the new epidermis to the underlying matrix (Clark *et al.*, 1982b), the fibrin and fibronectin provisional matrix dissipates (Clark *et al.*, 1982b), and the integrin ECM receptor expression markedly diminishes (Clark, 1990). Once a new stratified epidermis covers the wound surface the epidermal cells revert to their normal function.

Tissue remodelling is the final stage of wound repair; however, it greatly overlaps the preceding tissue formation stage. In fact as noted above, ECM remodelling as manifested by the re-establishment of basement membranes begins shortly after granulation tissue formation and re-epithelialization. ECM remodelling also occurs within the interstitial tissue. Most fibronectin is eliminated within a week or two after granulation tissue is established. Hyaluronate is replaced and/or supplemented with heparin sulphate proteoglycans in basement membrane regions and with dermatan/chondroitin sulphate proteoglycans in the interstitium. Type I collagen fibres are slowly remodelled to contain less type III collagen and to form large bundles that provide the residual scar with increasing tensile strength. After much ECM remodelling the easily traumatized granulation tissue slowly evolves into a strong mature scar.

REFERENCES

Ausprunk, D.H. and Folkman, J. (1977). Migration and proliferation of endothelial cells in preformed and newly formed blood vessels during tumor angiogenesis. *Microvasc. Res.*, **14**, 53–65.

Ausprunk, D.H., Boudreau, C.L. and Nelson, D.A. (1981). Proteoglycans in the microvasculature II. Histochemical localization in proliferating capillaries of the rabbit cornea. *Am. J. Pathol.*, **103**, 367–375.

Azizkhan, R.G., Azizkhan, J.C., Zetter, B.R. and Folkman, J. (1980). Mast cell heparin stimulates migration of capillary endothelial cells *in vitro. J. Exp. Med.*, **152**, 931–944.

Barrandon, Y. and Green, H. (1987). Cell migration is essential for sustained growth of keratinocyte colonies: the roles of transforming growth factor-α and epidermal growth factor. *Cell*, **50**, 1131–1137.

Carney, D.H. and Cunningham, D.D. (1978). Role of specific cell surface receptors in thrombin-stimulated cell division. *Cell*, **15**, 1341–1349.

Chien, S. (Ed.) (1989). *Vascular Endothelium in Health and Disease. Advances in Experimental Medicine and Biology.* Vol. 242. Plenum Press, New York.

Clark, R.A.F. (1990a). Cutaneous wound repair. In: Goldsmith, L.E. (Ed.), *Biochemistry and Physiology of the Skin*, Oxford University Press, Oxford.

Clark, R.A.F. (1990b). Fibronectin matrix deposition and fibronectin receptor expression in healing and normal skin. *J. Invest. Dermatol.*, in press.

Clark, R.A.F., Della Pelle, P., Manseau, E., Lanigan, J.M., Dvorak, H.F. and Colvin, R.B. (1982a). Blood vessel fibronectin increases in conjunction with endothelial cell proliferation and capillary ingrowth during wound healing. *J. Invest. Dermatol.*, **79**, 269–276.

Clark, R.A.F., Lanigan, J.M., Della Pelle, P., Manseau, E., Dvorak, H.F. and Colvin, R.B. (1982b). Fibronectin and fibrin provide a provisional matrix for epidermal cell migration during wound reepithelialization. *J. Invest. Dermatol.*, **79**, 264–269.

Clark, R.A.F., Folkford, J.M., Hart, C.E., Murray, M.J. and McPherson, J.M. (1989). Platelet-derived isoforms of PDGF stimulated fibroblasts to contraction collagen gel matrices. *J. Clin. Invest.*, **84**, 1036–1040.

Cohen, S. (1965). The stimulation of epidermal proliferation by a specific protein (EGF). *Dev. Biol.*, **12**, 394–407.

Derynck, R. (1988). Transforming growth factor-α. *Cell*, **54**, 593–595.

Folkman, J. and Klagsbrun, M. (1987). Angiogensic factors. *Science*, **235**, 442–447.

Furie, B. and Furie, B.C. (1988). The molecular basis of blood coagulation. *Cell*, **53**, 505–518.

Gabbiani, G., Chapponnier, C. and Huttner, I. (1978). Cytoplasmic filaments and gap junctions in epithelial cells and myofibroblasts during wound healing. *J. Cell Biol.*, **76**, 561–568.

Ginsberg, M.H., Loftus, J.C. and Plow, E.F. (1988). Cytoadhesins, integrins, and platelets. *Thromb. Haemost.*, **59**, 1–6.

Grimwood, R.E., Baskin, J.B. Nielsen, L.D., Ferris, C.F. and Clark, R.A.F. (1988). Fibronectin extracellular matrix assembly by human epidermal cells implanted into athymic mice. *J. Invest. Dermatol.*, **90**, 434–440.

Heino, J., Ignotz, R.A., Hemler, M.E., Crouse, C. and Massague, J. (1989). Regulation of cell adhesion receptors by transforming growth factor-β. Concomitant regulation of integrins that share a common β_1 subunit. *J. Biol. Chem.*, **264**, 380–388.

Ignotz, R.A., Heino, J. and Massague, J. (1989). Regulation of cell adhesion receptors by transforming growth factor-β. Regulation of vitronectin receptor and LFA-1. *J. Biol. Chem.*, **264**, 389–392.

Johnston, G.I., Cook, R.G. and McEver, R.P. (1989). Cloning of GMP-140, a granule membrane protein of platelets and endothelial cells: Sequence similarity to proteins involved in cell adhesion and inflammation. *Cell*, **56**, 1033–1044.

Madtes, D.K., Raines, E.W., Sakariassen, K.S., Assoian, R.K., Sporn, M.B., Bell, G.I. and Ross, R. (1988). Induction of transforming growth factor-α in activated human alveolar macrophages. *Cell*, **53**, 285–293.

Mauch, C., Hatamochi, A., Scharffetter, K. and Krieg, T. (1988). Regulation of collagen synthesis in fibroblasts within a three-dimensional collagen gel. *Exp. Cell Res.*, **178**, 493–503.

Mignatti, P., Tsuboi, R., Robbins, E. and Rifkin, D.B. (1989). *In vitro* angiogenesis on the human amniotic membrane: Requirement for basic fibroblast growth factor-induced proteinases. *J. Cell Biol.*, **108**, 671–682.

Nickoloff, B.J., Mitra, R.S., Riser, B.L., Dixit, V.M. and Varani, J. (1988). A modulation of keratinocyte motility. Correlation with production of extracellular matrix molecules in response to growth promoting and antiproliferative factors. *Am. J. Pathol.*, **132**, 543–551.

Riches, D.W.H. (1988). The multiple roles of macrophages in wound repair. In:

Clark, R.A.F. and Henson, P.M. (Eds), *Molecular and Cellular Biology of Wound Repair*, Plenum Press, New York, pp. 213–239.

Ross, R., Raines, E.W. and Bowen-Pope, D.F. (1986). The biology of platelet-derived growth factor. *Cell*, **46**, 155–169.

Ruoslahti, E. (1988). Fibronectin and its receptors. *Ann. Rev. Biochem.*, **57**, 375–413.

Shipley, G.D., Keeble, W.W., Hendrickson, J.E., Coffey, R.J. Jr and Pittelkow, M.R. (1989). Growth of normal human keratinocytes and fibroblasts in serum-free medium is stimulated by acidic and basic fibroblast growth factor. *J. Cell Physiol.*, **138**, 511–518.

Sporn, M.B., Roberts, A.B., Wakefield, L.M. and de Crombrugghe, B. (1987). Some recent advances in the chemistry and biology of transforming growth factor-beta. *J. Cell Biol.*, **105**, 1039–1045.

Terkeltaub, R.A. and Ginsberg, M.H. (1988). Platelets and response to injury. In: Clark, R.A.F. and Henson, P.M. (Eds), *Molecular and Cellular Biology of Wound Repair*, Plenum Press, New York, pp. 35–55.

Tonnesen, M.G. (1989). Neutrophil-endothelial cell interactions: mechanisms of neutrophil adherence to vascular endothelium. *J. Invest. Dermatol.*, **93**, 53S–58S.

Welch, M.P., Odland, G.F. and Clark, R.A.F. (1990). Temporal relationships between f-actin bundle formation, fibronectin and collagen assembly, fibronectin receptor expression, and wound contraction. *J. Cell Biol.*, **110**, 133–145.

Wikner, N.E., Baskin, J.B., Nielsen, L.D. and Clark, R.A.F. (1988). Transforming growth factor-β stimulates the expression of fibronectin by human keratinocytes. *J. Invest. Dermatol.*, **91**, 207–212.

Winter, G.D. (1962). Formation of the scab and the rate of epithelialization of superficial wounds in the skin of the young domestic pig. *Nature*, **193**, 293–294.

Molecular and Cellular Aspects of
Wound Repair

Wound Healing
Edited by H. Janssen, R. Rooman and J.I.S. Robertson
© 1991 Wrightson Biomedical Publishing Ltd

3

Regulation of Wound Healing by the T Cell-Dependent Immune System[*]

MARK C. REGAN and ADRIAN BARBUL

Departments of Surgery, Sinai Hospital and The Johns Hopkins Medical Institutions, Baltimore, Maryland, USA

Following injury the body restores tissue integrity via the process of wound healing, during which cellular elements and biochemical pathways interact in a complex manner to initiate, develop and terminate the reparative cascade. As our understanding of the healing process advances, the contribution of each cellular element and its interrelationship with the others becomes clearer. It is only relatively recently that the important role of the T cell-dependent immune system in wound healing has begun to be elucidated. Initially, a role for T lymphocytes in the process of tissue repair was inferred from *in vivo* studies which showed that lymphotrophic agents (i.e. growth hormone, vitamin A, arginine, and IL-2) lead to an increase in both wound breaking strength and wound reparative collagen deposition: conversely, lympholytic agents (i.e. steroids, cyclosporin A, retinoic acid, citral and chemotherapeutic agents) markedly impair wound fibroplasia (Barbul, 1988). In addition, nude rats which possess no or minimal T cell-dependent immune systems show diminished fibroblastic reaction in response to antigenic stimulation (Allen *et al.*, 1985). Since then further and more direct evidence for the participation of T cells in wound healing has accumulated.

HISTOLOGY

Following the influx of inflammatory cells, T lymphocytes migrate into wounds together with the macrophages. Numerically, macrophages out-number lymphocytes at all times during the healing process. In rats, wounds

*Supported by a grant from the National Institutes of Health, R29 GM 38650.

contain significantly more T lymphocytes in the deeper, reticular dermis portion of the wound 5 days post wounding when compared with 10 day old wounds. Similar, though less significant differences are observed in the superficial portion of the wound. Wound lymphocytic infiltration is a dynamic process, with populations of both T helper/effector and T suppressor/ cytotoxic lymphocytes being maximal in the superficial areas of the wound at 7 days (Fishel *et al.*, 1987).

Presently, there is no information regarding T cell activation at the site of normal repair. Available evidence suggests that T lymphocytes become functionally immunesuppressive at the wound site at about 7–10 days post-injury. Partially purified lymphocytes from rat sponge granulomas have been found to be unresponsive to either mitogens or IL-2 (Breslin *et al.*, 1988a). Additionally, they inhibit the normal thymic lymphocyte blastogenic response to plant lectins (Barbul *et al.*, 1983, 1984) and the growth of IL-2 dependent T cell clones to IL-2 (Breslin *et al.*, 1988b; Ford *et al.*, 1989). Wound lymphocytes constitutively secrete an immune inhibitory factor. This factor, present in wound fluid or in wound lymphocyte-conditioned medium, appears 7–10 days post wounding, suggesting that the wound environment activates and programmes wound infiltrating lymphocytes for this immune-suppressive function. The inhibitory effect appears to be specific to lymphocyte lines since proliferation of 3T3 fibroblasts is not affected. The lymphokine(s) responsible for this activity remains unidentified but has been partially characterized. It has a molecular weight >50 kDa and appears to be a protein precipitable with trichloroacetic acid or ammonium chloride. It is heat resistant at 56°C for 60 min and trypsin resistant but neuraminidase sensitive.

PARTICIPATION OF LYMPHOKINES IN WOUND HEALING

In vitro activity of lymphokines

Numerous lymphocyte secretory products (lymphokines) have been shown to affect *in vitro* fibroblast migration, replication and protein synthesis (Table 1). Both inhibitory and stimulatory factors have been described. However, little is known about the actual *in vivo* presence of such factors in wounds and even less is understood about their possible interaction.

Presence of lymphokines in wounds

The *in vivo* regulation of wound healing almost certainly involves a complex multi-factorial interaction of cytokines derived from T lymphocytes, monocytes and other elements in the local micro-environment. It seems reasonable to suppose that wound fibroblast activity is the end result of the

Table 1.   Effect of various lymphokines on *in vitro* fibroblast activity (adapted and updated from Barbul 1989b).

	Proliferation	Chemotaxis	Collagen Synthesis
LDCF-F		↑	
FIF		↓	
FAF	↑		↑
IF	↓		
γ-IFN	↓ ↑		↓
α-IFN		↓	
TGF-β	↑ ↓	↑	↑
LT	↑		↑
CPF			↑

Key: LDCF-F, lymphocyte-derived chemotactic factor for fibroblasts; FIF, fibroblast inhibitory factor; FAF, fibroblast activating factor; IF, inhibition factor; γ-IFN, γ-interferon; α-IFN, α-interferon; TGF-β, transforming growth factor-β; LT, lymphotoxin; CPF, collagen production factor.

various factors acting in sequence and/or in concert, with each cytokine modulating the effect of others.

One method of studying the role of wound lymphocytes in wound healing is to detect biologically active lymphokines in the wound environment and to demonstrate both *in vitro* and *in vivo* regulatory functions for such lymphokines. Transforming growth factor-β (TGF-β) is a potent fibroblast (Postlethwaite *et al.*, 1987) and macrophage chemotactic agent (Wahl *et al.*, 1986) *in vitro*. Although antigenically TGF-β is present in large quantities at the wound site, biological activity of this moiety has not been demonstrated (Cromack *et al.*, 1987). Ford *et al.* (1989) have demonstrated the presence of biologically active IL-1, TNF-α and IL-6 at various times post-injury in murine wound fluid, with the highest concentrations present during the first 3 days following wounding, at a time when neutrophils are the predominant cell population. Other lymphokines such as γ-interferon (γ-IFN) have not been demonstrated to be present in 10 day old wound fluid (Lazarou *et al.*, 1989).

In vivo effect of lymphokines on wound healing

Roberts *et al.* (1986) have shown that subcutaneous injection of 800 μg of TGF-β into newborn mice resulted in increased granulation tissue formation. Application of TGF-β to linear incisions in rats leads to increased wound breaking strength and collagen deposits with a concomitant rise in mononuclear cell and fibroblast infiltration in both normal and steroid-treated animals (Mustoe, 1987; Pierce, 1989). Administration of human recombinant IL-2 (60 000 U/day and 14 000 U/day) to rats also significantly augmented fresh and fixed wound breaking strengths with a parallel rise in wound reparative collagen as assessed by the hydroxyproline content of subcutaneously implanted polyvinyl alcohol sponges (Barbul et al., 1986).

On the other hand, implantation of subcutaneous osmotic pumps containing γ-IFN into mice resulted in decreased thickness and collagen content of the fibrous capsule that forms around the pumps (Granstein et al., 1987). Furthermore, systemic γ-IFN administration also impairs inflammation and collagen synthesis (Granstein et al., 1989).

EFFECT OF T CELL IMMUNE MANIPULATION ON WOUND HEALING

Role of the thymus

Adult thymectomy in rats leads to increased wound maturation without increased collagen synthesis. This effect is reversed by intraperitoneal placement of autologous thymic grafts contained in Millipore chambers (Barbul et al., 1982). Since adult thymectomy prevents induction of T suppressor cells, it was postulated that these cell subtypes may normally down-regulate the wound healing process. In mice, the in vivo administration of purified or synthetic active fractions of thymic hormones (thymulin, thymopentin, and thymosin fraction V) in doses known to have full immunological activity impairs wound healing, as assessed by both wound breaking strength and the hydroxyproline content of subcutaneously implanted polyvinyl alcohol sponges (Barbul et al., 1989a). Since the administered thymic hormones induce T suppressor cell differentation and maturation, these findings lend support to the hypothesis that T suppressor lymphocytes are responsible for the observed inhibition of wound healing.

In vivo role of lymphocytes

One method of determining the in vivo role of lymphocytes in wound healing is to study the effect of lymphocyte depletion on the fibroplastic process. Two early in vivo studies involving lymphocyte depletion noted no effect on wound healing (Stein and Levenson, 1966; Scott and Phillips, 1969). In these studies the source, efficacy and dosing of the anti-lymphocyte serum were not clearly stated and in one study the wounds were examined prior to the fibroblastic phase of healing.

In our laboratory we have studied the effect of global T cell depletion in mice by using specific monoclonal antibodies. The intraperitoneal injection of 1 mg of a rat anti-mouse (IgG_{2b}) cytotoxic monoclonal antibody ($30H_{12}$) active against the Thy 1.2 (all T) determinant achieved >95% Thy 1.2 cell depletion in both peripheral blood and spleen at 24 hours. T cell depletion was maintained by weekly injection of the monoclonal antibody and ranged at death from 95–57% in peripheral blood and 86–68% in spleen. Wound healing was assessed at 2,3 and 4 weeeks by wound breaking strength and the hydroxyproline content of sponge granulomas. Both wound breaking strength and wound collagen deposition were significantly impaired (Fig. 1) (Peterson et al., 1987).

Depletion of T helper/effector cells alone using the cytotoxic monoclonal antibody GK1.5, reactive against the L3T4 antigen (CD4) in mice achieved depletions of 79.8% at 24 hours to 65% at 4 weeks in peripheral blood and 70.4% to 57.2% in spleens with a parallel decrease in Thy 1.2 (all T) marker bearing cells. However, no effect on either wound breaking strength or wound collagen deposition was observed. In contrast depletion of the T suppressor/cytotoxic lymphocyte subset using the 2.43 monoclonal antibody which is reactive against the Lyt 2 antigen (CD8), caused marked enhancement in wound healing at 2 and 4 weeks post-wounding. Depletion ranged from 93.4% at 24 hours to 94.1% at 4 weeks in peripheral blood and 94.8–86.5%, respectively in spleen (Fig. 2) (Barbul et al., 1989b).

Thus, it would appear that T suppressor/cytotoxic cells have an inhibitory effect on wound healing and their in vivo depletion up to 14 days following wounding significantly enhances wound fibroplasia. As global depletion of T lymphocytes had significantly impaired wound fibroplasia, it was expected that depletion of either the helper or suppressor subset could duplicate these findings. However, depletion of the T helper/effector subset had no effect on wound healing. This could be due to the relative increase in T suppressor/cytotoxic cells following T helper/effector depletion, which may have abrogated any effect that the use of GK1.5 might have had on healing. Considering the finding that there is a heavy infiltration of activated T helper lymphocytes (CD4) in the presence of abnormal healing, as evidenced by excessive fibrosis or granuloma formation (Allen et al., 1985; Wahl and Malone, 1985, 1986), an enhancer role may yet be demonstrated for T helper/effector cells despite a failure to substantiate this to date.

Further support of this work comes from studies of wound healing in the congenitally athymic nude mouse (Barbul et al., 1989c). These animals have a profoundly impaired T cell dependent system and demonstrate significantly enhanced wound breaking strength when compared with normal thymus bearing animals. This is accompanied by a marked increase in the amount of reparative collagen synthesized at the wound site as assessed by the hydroxyproline content of sponge granulomas (Fig. 3). Administration of the

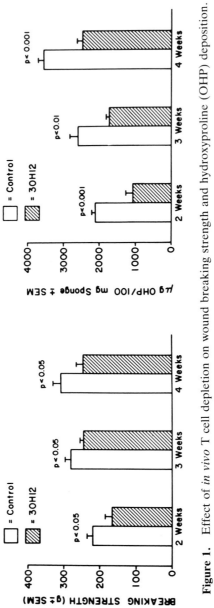

Figure 1.   Effect of *in vivo* T cell depletion on wound breaking strength and hydroxyproline (OHP) deposition.

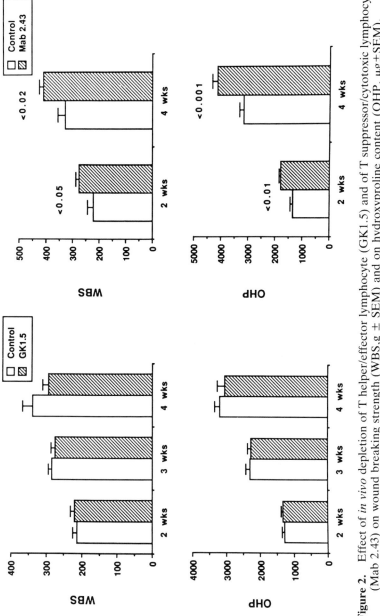

Figure 2. Effect of *in vivo* depletion of T helper/effector lymphocyte (GK1.5) and of T suppressor/cytotoxic lymphocyte (Mab 2.43) on wound breaking strength (WBS,g ± SEM) and on hydroxyproline content (OHP, µg±SEM).

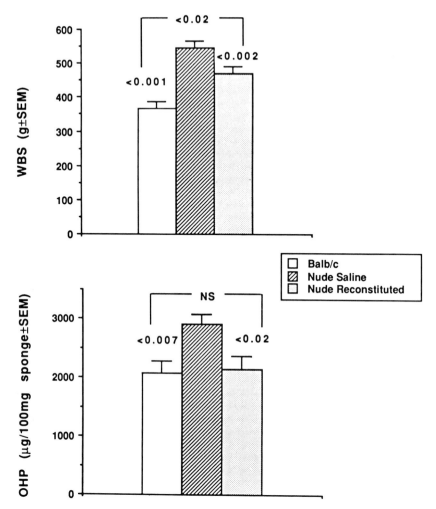

Figure 3. Wound healing parameters in normal, athymic and athymic T cell-reconstituted mice (WBS, wound breaking strength; OHP, hydroxyproline).

all T, anti-Thy 1.2 ($30H_{12}$) monoclonal antibody in order to deplete small numbers of extra thymically derived T cells which are present in such animals, had no effect on wound fibroplasia but confirmed the previously observed significant decrease in wound breaking strength and hydroxyproline content when administered to normal control mice. T cell reconstitution of nude mice, sufficient to induce delayed type hypersensitivity responses and confirmed by FACS analysis of peripheral blood and spleens, resulted in a significant decrease in wound breaking strength and hydroxyproline content in the nude animals, towards the levels observed in normal Balb/c controls (Fig. 3).

On the basis of the foregoing evidence one might therefore speculate that the T cells have a facilitatory effect on wound healing early in the process. Their main effect however, mediated by the Ts/c subset, appears to be down-regulation of the exuberant cellular activation that occurs early in the healing process.

CONCLUSIONS

The presence of T lymphocytes at the site of wound healing is well established. It is evident that T lymphocytes are necessary for the usual progression and orderly outcome of normal wound healing. However wound healing can be initiated and progress in the absence of T lymphocytes. Thus the role of the T lymphocyte appears to be mainly in moderating and orchestrating the debridement and repair process. Activated T lymphocytes are capable of recruiting, expanding and activating the fibroblasts which are primarily responsible for this repair process. This control may be achieved via lymphokines acting either directly on the fibroblasts or via the mediation of macrophages or both. Resident macrophages are suppresive of fibroblast function, while activated macrophages are stimulatory. Early in the course of wound healing T helper/effector cells may promote macrophage activity. The T helper/effector cells are activated in turn by, among other factors, antigen presented by the macrophages thus providing a positive feedback loop. As antigen is cleared this cycle is down-regulated; however, in abnormal circumstances with continued antigenic load, stimulation of the T helper activity is maintained and the macrophages continue to be stimulatory to fibroblast activity.

Under normal circumstances this T helper/effector mediated stimulation may be overwhelmed quickly by the suppressive influence of the T suppressor/cytotoxic lymphocytes, which are proportionately much increased over resting levels, with a resulting tendency to down-regulate the system towards resting states and hence terminate the process of wound healing in an orderly manner.

In addition, the T lymphocytes exhibit an autocrine self regulation, as evidenced by suppression of mitogenesis in the wound environment which may prevent the generation of autoreactive T cell clones in response to self antigens. Thus there seems to be a well-defined balance between stimulatory and inhibitory T lymphocyte influences on wound cellular activity. Our present knowledge of how this balance is achieved is limited, but it is clear than an imbalance could result in wound failure or conversely in excessive fibrosis.

REFERENCES

Allen, J.B., Malone, D.G., Wahl, S.M. *et al.* (1985). Role of the thymus in streptococcal cell wall-induced arthritis and hepatic granuloma formation. *J. Clin. Invest.*, **46**, 1042–1056.

Barbul, A. (1988). Role of the T cell-dependent immune system in wound healing. *Prog. Clin. Biol. Res.*, **266**, 161–175.

Barbul, A. (1989). Immune regulation of wound healing. In: Faist, E., Green D.R. and Ninnemann, J. (eds), *Immune Consequences of Trauma, Shock and Sepsis*, Springer Verlag, Berlin, pp. 339–49.

Barbul, A., Sisto, D.A., Rettura, G. *et al.* (1982). Thymic inhibition of wound healing: Abrogation by adult thymectomy. *J. Surg. Res.*, **32**, 338–342.

Barbul, A., Rettura, G., Levenson, S.M. *et al.* (1983). Fluid and mononuclear cells from healing wounds inhibit thymocyte immune-responsiveness. *J. Surg. Res.*, **34**, 505–509.

Barbul, A., Fishel, R.S., Shimazu, S. *et al.* (1984). Inhibition of host immunity by fluid and mononuclear cells from healing wounds. *Surgery*, **96**, 315–320.

Barbul, A., Knud-Hansen, J., Wasserkrug, H.L. *et al.* (1986). Interleukin 2 enhances wound healing in rats. *J. Surg. Res.*, **40**, 315–319.

Barbul, A., Shaw, T., Frankel, H. *et al.* (1989a). Inhibition of wound repair by thymic hormones. *Surgery*, **106**, 373–377.

Barbul, A., Breslin, R.J., Woodyard, J.P. *et al.* (1989b). The effect of *in vivo* T helper and T suppressor lymphocyte depletion on wound healing. *Ann. Surg.*, **209**, 479–483.

Barbul, A., Shawe, T., Rotter, S.M. *et al.* (1989c). Wound healing in nude mice: A study on the regulatory role of lymphocytes in fibroplasia. *Surgery*, **105**, 764–769.

Breslin, R.J., Wasserkrug, H.L. and Efron, G. (1988a). Suppressor cell generation during normal wound healing. *J. Surg. Res.*, **44**, 321–325.

Breslin, R.J., Barbul, A. and Kupper, T.S. (1988b). Generation of an anti-IL2 factor in healing wounds. *Arch. Surg.*, **123**, 305–308.

Cromack, D.T., Sporn, M.B., Roberts, A.B. *et al.* (1987). Transforming growth factor-β levels in rat wound chambers. *J. Surg. Res.*, **42**, 622–628.

Fishel, R.S., Barbul, A., Beschorner, W.E. *et al.* (1987). Lymphocyte participation in wound healing: Morphologic assessment using monoclonal antibodies. *Ann. Surg.*, **206**, 25–29.

Ford, H.R., Hoffman, R.A., Wing, E.J. *et al.* (1989). Wound cytokines in the sponge matrix model. *Arch. Surg.*, **124**, 1422–1428.

Granstein, R.D., Murphy, G.F., Margolis, R.J. *et al.* (1987). Gamma-interferon inhibits collagen synthesis *in vivo* in the mouse. *J. Clin. Invest.*, **79**, 1254–1258.

Granstein, R.D., Deak, M.R., Jacques, S.L. *et al.* (1989). The systemic administration of gamma interferon inhibits collagen synthesis and acute inflammation in a murine skin wounding model. *J. Invest. Dermatol.*, **93**, 18–27.

Lazarou, S.A., Barbul, A., Wasserkrug, H.L. *et al.* (1989). The wound is a possible source of post-traumatic immunesuppression. *Arch. Surg.*, **124**, 1429–1431.

Mustoe, T.A., Pierce, G.F., Thomason, *et al.* (1987). Accelerated healing of incisional wounds in rats induced by transforming growth factor-β. *Science*, **237**, 1333–1336.

Peterson, J.M., Barbul, A., Breslin, R.J. *et al.* (1987). Significance of T lymphocytes in wound healing. *Surgery*, **102**, 300–305.

Pierce, G.F., Mustoe, T.A., Lingelbach, J. *et al.* (1989). Transforming growth factor-β reverses the glucorticoid-induced wound-healing deficit in rats: Possible regulation in macrophages by platelet-derived growth factor. *Proc. Natl Acad. Sci. USA*, **86**, 2229–2233.

Postlethwaite, A.E., Keski-Oja, J., Moses, H.L. *et al.* (1987). Stimulation of the chemotactic migration of human fibroblasts by transforming growth factor beta. *J. Exp. Med.*, **165**, 251–256.

Roberts, A.B., Sporn, M.B., Assoian, R.K. *et al.* (1986). Transforming growth factor type β: Rapid induction of fibrosis and angiogenesis *in vivo* and stimulation of collagen formation *in vitro*. *Proc. Natl Acad. Sci. USA*, **83**, 4167–4171.

Scott, R.A.P. and Phillips, B. (1969). The effect of anti-lymphocyte serum on wound healing. *Brit. J. Surg.*, **56**, 700 (abstract 119).

Stein, J.M. and Levenson, S.M. (1966). Effect of the inflammatory reaction on subsequent wound healing. *Surg. Forum*, **17**, 484–485.

Wahl, S.M. and Malone, D.G. (1985). Spontaneous production of fibroblast-activating factors by synovial inflammatory cells. *J. Exp. Med.*, **161**, 210–222.

Wahl, S.M., Hunt, D.A., Allen, J.B. *et al.* (1986). Bacterial cell wall-induced hepatic granulomas: An *in vivo* model of T cell-dependent fibrosis. *J. Exp. Med.*, **163**, 884–902.

Wound Healing
Edited by H. Janssen, R. Rooman and J.I.S. Robertson

4

Cytokine Regulation of Collagen Metabolism During Wound Healing *in vitro* and *in vivo*

M. KULOZIK, M. HECKMANN, C. MAUCH, K. SCHARFFETTER
and TH. KRIEG

Dermatology Clinic of the Ludwig Maximilians University, Munich, Germany

ABSTRACT

Collagen metabolism is closely controlled during repair processes. Exact regulation is achieved by the interaction of fibroblasts with the surrounding extracellular matrix as well as by cytokines known to regulate specifically collagen gene expression and collagen metabolism. We used cDNA probes specific for collagen types I, III, VI and collagenase to investigate the influence of γ-interferon (γ-IFN), tumour necrosis factor-α (TNF-α) and transforming growth factor-β (TGF-β) *in vitro*. In addition, *in situ* hybridization studies were carried out in order to obtain information about the regulation of collagen gene expression in the tissue during primary and secondary wound healing, and also in fibroblasts grown in three-dimensional collagen lattices. The studies indicate that synthesis of collagen I and III is strongly induced at a pretranslational level in early phases of wound healing following injury of the skin. This is followed by tightly controlled down-regulation of collagen. *In vitro*, a combination of γ-IFN and TNF-α resulted in a strong reduction of collagen gene expression indicating that these cytokines may play a role during wound healing. Similarly, a close contact of fibroblasts with the surrounding collagen fibrils reduces gene expression of collagens I and III but not collagen VI. Comparison of *in vitro* and *in vivo* data using *in situ* hybridization might help to obtain more information about the complex regulatory events resulting in a physiological repair process.

INTRODUCTION

Wound healing is defined as a highly regulated sequence of various cellular events leading to a reconstitution of the integrity of a tissue following injury (Clark, 1985). Although the biological significance of many of these events is still unknown, *de novo* biosynthesis of collagen, the major structural component of the dermis, plays a central role during restoration of cutaneous tissue defects (Clore *et al.*, 1979; Kurkinen *et al.*, 1980; Scharffetter *et al.*, 1989b). The exact regulation of collagen metabolism is achieved by the interaction of fibroblasts with the surrounding extracellular matrix as well as by cytokines released from platelets, endothelial cells and inflammatory cells.

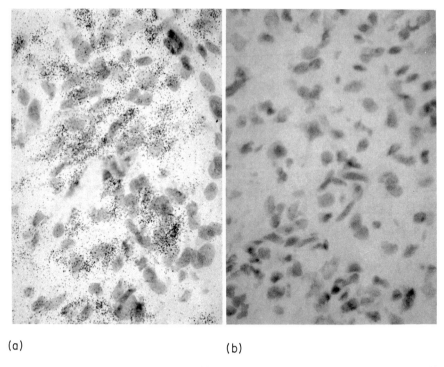

(a)   (b)

Figure 1. Localization of collagen α1(I) chain mRNA synthesizing cells in a 6 day old granulation tissue. Intense labelling of fibroblastic cells within newly formed tissue. Labelling with the collagen α1(I) antisense RNA probe (a). No labelling is seen with the α1(I) sense RNA probe which serves as a negative control (b). Magnification × 250 (reproduced with permission, from Scharffetter *et al.*, 1989b.)

LOCALIZATION OF COLLAGEN GENE EXPRESSION DURING WOUND HEALING BY *IN SITU* HYBRIDIZATION

In situ hybridization techniques using a probe for collagen α1(I) were used to study the localization of collagen gene expressing fibroblasts in tissue sections taken from consecutive stages of wound healing. Only 16–24 hours after the initial damage distinct labelling was seen in fibroblastic cells in the deep dermis (Scharffetter *et al.*, 1989b) (Fig. 1). After 8 days, when a granulation tissue had been formed, most of the intensely labelled fibroblasts were found directly beneath the newly reconstituted epidermis, whereas only a few cells located in the deep dermis were labelled (Fig. 2). This pattern was even more

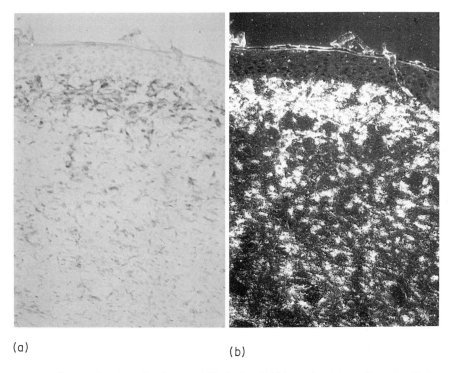

(a)

(b)

Figure 2. Localization of collagen α1(I) chain mRNA synthesizing cells at day 8 after initial wounding in (a) bright and (b) dark field microscopy. Most of the highly labelled cells are found directly below the epidermis and only weak labelling is seen in the deep dermis. Procedure as in Fig. 1. Magnification × 75. (reproduced with permission, from Scharffetter *et al.*, 1989b.)

prominent by days 13–21, where densely labelled fibroblasts were exclusively localized directly beneath the epidermis. Twenty-six days after wounding no labelled cells were detected, indicating that *de novo* biosynthesis of collagen during dermal repair had almost been completed. These data demonstrate that collagen α1(I) chain gene expression is strictly controlled during wound healing. It is induced and down-regulated in very distinct areas in a time-dependent fashion.

At present, our understanding of the mechanisms inducing and reducing collagen synthesis under these conditions is limited. In early stages during the inflammatory phase many biologically active mediators, e.g. TGF-β, platelet-derived growth factor (PDGF), etc., are released, which can stimulate collagen production. This release will cease later on and other mediators can selectively inhibit collagen gene expression.

THE INFLUENCE OF MEDIATORS ON COLLAGEN METABOLISM

Most information concerning the regulation of collagen metabolism by cytokines has been obtained from *in vitro* studies and little is known about their role *in vivo*. Cytokines are released by a variety of different cell types during various stages of wound healing where they probably act together in a complex concert and the actual metabolic control of tissue events depends on the relative concentration of individual cytokines. TGF-β as well as IL-1 have been found to induce collagen synthesis in fibroblasts at a pretranslational level (Ignotz and Massague, 1986; Postlethwaite *et al.*, 1988). On the other hand, decreased synthesis of collagen I and III is seen after incubating fibroblasts with γ-interferon. This effect is also accompanied by diminished steady-state levels of the corresponding mRNAs due to decreased gene transcription (Czaja *et al.*, 1987). It seems to be highly specific since fibronectin synthesis is not influenced by γ-IFN and not every type of collagen is regulated in the same way. While the interstitial collagens I and III are reduced at the transcriptional level, collagen VI is regulated via mRNA reduction of only one subunit (Heckmann *et al.*, 1989). Tumour necrosis factor-α (TNF-α) also reduces collagen synthesis, induces collagenase gene expression and acts synergistically with γ-IFN in reducing collagen synthesis (Scharffetter *et al.*, 1989a). So combined activity of these cytokines might be responsible for the effective down-regulation of collagen gene expression in later stages of wound healing.

THE INFLUENCE OF THE EXTRACELLULAR MATRIX

The extracellular matrix is composed of a large variety of multidomain molecules (Hay, 1983). Initially, it was assumed that these represent the structurally stable material surrounding fibroblasts; there is now growing evidence that the extracellular matrix (ECM) not only acts as the structural scaffold of the tissue but can also provide signals for cells, thus controlling several cellular functions.

So, the growth of fibroblasts is reduced when the cells are embedded in a three-dimensional collagen matrix (Mauch *et al.*, 1988). Contact of fibroblasts with mature collagen I fibrils leads to a reduction of collagen synthesis and to an activation of collagenase gene expression (Mauch *et al.*, 1989). In addition, collagen synthesis in fibroblasts underlies a feedback regulation. Interstitial collagens are synthesized in a precursor form, procollagen, containing two large procollagen peptides located at each end. After secretion of the molecules into the extracellular space the procollagen peptides are cleaved off by two specific proteases. Both procollagen peptides have been shown to act as feedback inhibitors and to control collagen synthesis.

An increased cleavage rate leading to high amounts of free peptides has been observed in fibroblasts cultured within a dense connective tissue network (Mauch *et al.*, 1988). Under these conditions collagen synthesis is rapidly down-regulated, which could be due to either the close contact of the cells to the three-dimensional collagen fibrils or the high amount of free procollagen peptides (Mauch and Krieg, 1990).

CONCLUSION

Connective tissue formation and remodelling during wound healing represent a highly ordered sequence of events finally leading to restoration of the tissue. In early stages fibroblastic cells within a loose connective tissue matrix are attracted by mediators like TGF-β and IL-1, which are released from inflammatory cells, endothelial cells and platelets. This is then followed by a down-regulation of collagen gene expression which first occurs in the lower dermis. After 10–13 days only cells located beneath the newly formed basement membrane are still actively synthesizing collagen. *In vitro* data suggest that this decrease is mediated by two mechanisms. The close interaction of fibroblasts with the surrounding dense connective tissue matrix results in a reduction of collagen synthesis and at the same time in an induction of collagenase gene expression as well as the activation of the synthesized enzyme. In addition, concomitant release of γ-IFN and TNF-α which act synergistically can markedly affect collagen gene expression in fibroblasts. Probably both the increasing density of the surrounding extracellular matrix and a change in the release of mediators can control the reprogramming of activated fibroblasts during later phases of wound healing at a local level (Fig. 3). Further studies of the molecular mechanism of these

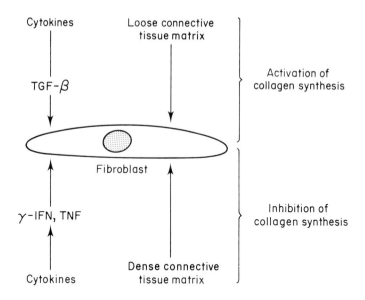

Figure 3. Schematic drawing of the regulation of fibroblast metabolic activity by various mediators and the connective tissue matrix.

cell–cell and cell–matrix interactions are essential in order to understand these physiological repair mechanisms and to develop new therapeutic strategies to modulate wound healing.

REFERENCES

Clark, R.A.F. (1985). Cutaneous tissue repair: Basic biological considerations. *J. Am. Acad. Dermatol.*, **13**, 701–725.

Clore, J.W., Cohen, J.K. and Diegelmann, R.F. (1979). Quantitation of collagen types I and III during wound healing in rat skin. *Proc. Soc. Exp. Biol. Med.*, **161**, 337–340.

Czaja, M.J. Weiner, F.R., Eghbali, M., Giambrone, M.A., Eghbali, M. and Zern, M. (1987). Differential effects of interferon-gamma on collagen and fibronectin gene expression. *J. Biol. Chem.*, **262**, 13348–13351.

Hay, E.D. (1983). *Cell Biology of the Extracellular Matrix*, Plenum Press, New York.

Heckmann, M., Aumailley, M., Hatamochi, A., Chu, M.L., Timpl, R. and Krieg, Th. (1989). Down regulation of $\alpha 3(VI)$ chain expression by interferon-gamma decreases synthesis and deposition of collagen VI. *Eur. J. Biochem.*, **182**, 719–726.

Ignotz, R.A. and Massague, J. (1986). Transforming growth factor-β stimulates the expression of fibronectin and collagen and their incorporation into the extracellular matrix. *J. Biol. Chem.*, **261**, 4337–4342.

Kurkinen, M., Vaheri, A., Roberts, P.J. and Stenan, S. (1980). Sequential appearance of fibronectin and collagen in experimental granulation tissue. *Lab. Invest.*, **43**, 47–51.

Mauch, C. and Krieg, Th. (1990). Fibroblast–matrix interactions and their role in the pathogenesis of fibrosis. *Rheum. Dis. Clinics N. Am.*, **16**, 93–107.

Mauch, C., Hatamochi, A., Scharffetter, K. and Krieg, Th. (1988). Regulation of collagen synthesis in fibroblasts within a three-dimensional collagen gel. *Exp. Cell Res.*, **178**, 493–530.

Mauch, C., Adelmann-Grill, B., Hatamochi, A. and Krieg, Th. (1989). Collagenase gene expression in fibroblasts is regulated by a three-dimensional contact with collagen. *FEBS Letters*, **250**, 301–305.

Postlethwaite, A.E., Raghow, R., Stricklin, G.P., Poppleton, A., Seyer, J.M. and Kang, A.H. (1988). Modulation of fibroblast function by interleukin-I increased steady-state accumulation of type I procollagen mRNA and stimulation of other functions but not chemotaxis by human recombinant interleukin-1 α and β. *J. Cell Biol.*, **106**, 311–318.

Scharffetter, K., Heckmann, M., Hatamochi, A., Mauch, C., Stein, B., Riethmüller, G., Ziegler-Heitbrock, H.B. and Krieg, Th. (1989a). Synergistic effect of tumour necrosis factor-α and interferon-gamma on collagen synthesis of human fibroblasts *in vitro*. *Exp. Cell Res.*, **181**, 409–419.

Scharffetter, K., Kulozik, M., Stolz, W., Lankat-Buttgereit, B., Hatamochi, A., Söhnchen, R. and Krieg, Th. (1989b). Localization of collagen α1(I) gene expression during wound healing by *in situ* hybridization. *J. Invest. Dermatol.*, **93**, 405–412.

Wound Healing
Edited by H. Janssen, R. Rooman and J.I.S. Robertson
© 1991 Wrightson Biomedical Publishing Ltd

5

The Role of Fibroblast Growth Factors in Wound Healing in the Central Nervous System

SETH P. FINKLESTEIN[1,3] CORNELIO G. CADAY[1,3] and MICHAEL KLAGSBRUN[2,4,5]

[1]CNS Growth Factor Research Laboratory, Massachusetts General Hospital, Boston, [2]Children's Hospital Medical Center, Boston, and Departments of [3]Neurology, [4]Surgery, and [5]Biological Chemistry, Harvard Medical School, Boston, Massachusetts, USA

Although complete wound healing, as such, does not occur in the mature mammalian central nervous system (CNS), a process of cellular events does occur that results in the repair of damaged tissue and the partial restoration of neurological function after injury. Head trauma and stroke are common causes of focal brain injury in humans (Adams and Victor, 1985). Following such injury, there is disruption of the 'blood–brain barrier' and infiltration of circulating blood phagocytes into wounds, occurring within hours to days (Adams and Sidman, 1982). These early reactions are followed by the proliferation of glial cells and blood vessels ('neovascularization') at the borders of wounds, occurring within the first few weeks after injury (du Bois et al., 1985). These changes contribute to the removal of cellular debris, and to the restoration of the structural integrity of tissue. Finally, focal CNS wounds are accompanied by sprouting of some neural fibre types occurring within weeks to months after injury. Although full regrowth of severed axons does not occur in the mature mammalian CNS, local sprouting of injured axons and collateral sprouting of other axons into denervated synapses does occur over short distances (Cotman and Nieto-Sampedro, 1984). Such sprouting has been correlated with functional recovery in several model systems (Azmitia et al., 1978; Cotman and Nieto-Sampedro, 1984).

Abundant evidence links the actions of macromolecular growth factors to the process of wound healing in skin, bone, and other peripheral tissues (Davidson et al., 1985; Gospodarowicz et al., 1987; Klagsbrun, 1990). By analogy, growth factors are likely to play an equally important role in wound

41

healing in the CNS. In this regard, fibroblast growth factors (FGFs) are of particular interest, since both forms, acidic and basic, are found in relatively high concentrations in the mammalian CNS, and have potent multipotential trophic effects on CNS cells *in vitro*. Both acidic FGF (aFGF) and basic FGF (bFGF) are potent *gliotrophic* agents that promote the survival and proliferation of CNS glial cells (Pettman *et al.*, 1985). Both are potent *angiogenic* factors that promote endothelial cell proliferation *in vitro*, and capillary proliferation *in vivo* (Folkman and Klagsbrun, 1987). Finally, both aFGF and bFGF are potent *neuronotrophic* factors that support the survival and outgrowth of a wide variety of CNS neurons in culture (Walicke, 1988). Indeed, FGFs have a wider spectrum of action on CNS cells in general (and on CNS neurons in particular) than any other characterized brain growth factor.

Because of these multipotential effects on CNS cells, FGFs are likely to play an important role in the cascade of cellular reactions that characterizes wound healing in the CNS. We have investigated the role of FGFs in models of both mechanical and ischaemic brain injury (stroke) in the mature rodent brain (Finklestein *et al.*, 1988; 1989a; b; 1990). In initial studies, focal mechanical (suction) lesions were made in the lateral cerebral cortex of mature Sprague–Dawley rats. At one week after injury, animals were sacrificed, brains were removed, and regions surrounding lesions (c. 300 mg tissue) were taken for FGF assay. Homologous regions were taken from the intact rat brain as controls. Brain tissue was homogenized in 1.0 M NaCl, 100 mM Tris-HCL, pH 7.5, and centrifuged, and the supernatant was removed for assay.

FGFs are commonly assayed by mitogenic activity on Balb/c 3T3 cells *in vitro*, and are unique among characterized 3T3 mitogens by virtue of their strong binding to heparin (Klagsbrun, 1990). In our studies, FGFs were assayed in brain tissue homogenates by heparin-affinity chromatography coupled to Balb/c 3T3 mitogenic assay (Finklestein *et al.*, 1989a; b; 1990). In initial studies, an equivalent amount of total protein from intact or injured brain was loaded onto a heparin-sepharose affinity column. The column was washed with buffer containing 0.1 M NaCl, and retained proteins were eluted with a continuous gradient of 0.1–3.0 M NaCl in buffer. Eluted fractions were assayed for ability to stimulate ^{3}H-thymidine incorporation into DNA of Balb/c 3T3 cells *in vitro* (Fig. 1). Consistent with previous results, we found that most of the 3T3 mitogenic activity in brain homogenates bound tightly to heparin-affinity columns, and was eluted at 1.0–2.0 M NaCl, a position characteristic for FGFs (Klagsbrun and Shing, 1985). Moreover, given an equivalent amount of total protein loaded onto the column, we found a marked increase in 3T3 stimulatory activity in homogenates from the injured v. intact brain (Fig. 1).

The presence of FGFs in peaks eluted from heparin-sepharose affinity

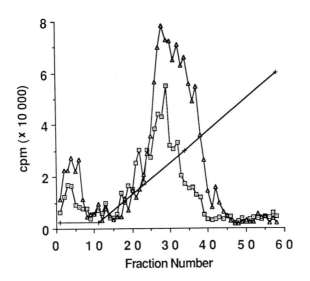

Figure 1. Heparin-affinity chromatography of homogenates from injured v. intact brain. An equivalent amount of total protein (c. 45 mg) in homogenates from injured (triangle symbols) or intact (square symbols) rat brain was loaded on to a heparin-sepharose affinity column, which was washed with buffer containing 0.1 M NaCl. Retained proteins were eluted with a continuous gradient of 0.1–3.0 M NaCl (solid line). Fractions were assayed for ability to stimulate ^{3}H-thymidine incorporation into Balb/c 3T3 cells (expressed as cpm). A marked increase in heparin-bound mitogenic activity was found in homogenates from injured v. intact brain.

columns was shown by immuno- (Western) blotting using specific anti-FGF sera. Fractions under peaks of mitogenic activity were pooled, lyophilized, electrophoresced on 15% SDS–PAGE gels, electroblotted onto nitrocellulose, and stained with specific anti-FGF sera. These polyclonal antisera were raised against non-homologous peptide sequences of either aFGF or bFGF and react appropriately and specifically with these factors on Western blots (Wadzinski *et al.*, 1987). Figure 2 shows a blot stained with anti-bFGF sera. This antibody stained a bovine bFGF but not aFGF standard (Fig. 2, lane 1 v. 2; 18 v. 16 kDa, respectively), and detected three bands of bFGF immunoreactivity in rat brain homogenate (Fig. 2, lanes 3 and 4; 18, 22, and 24 kDa). These results are consistent with those of other investigators, who have reported similar higher molecular weight forms of bFGF in rodent brain (Moscatelli *et al.*, 1987). Moreover, consistent with the results of the mitogenic assay (Fig. 1), we found a marked increase in bFGF immunoreactivity in fractions from injured v. intact brain (Fig. 2, lane 3 v. 4, respectively). Basic FGF immunoreactivity was appropriately abolished by pre-incubation of antisera with an excess of peptide immunogen (Fig. 2, lanes

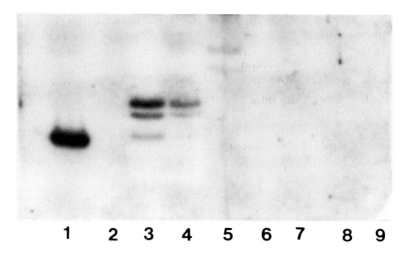

1   2   3   4   5   6   7   8   9

Figure 2. Western blot characterization of homogenates from injured v. intact brain. Fractions under peaks eluted from heparin-sepharose affinity column (Fig. 1) were pooled, concentrated, electrophoresed on 15% SDS–PAGE gels, and blotted on to nitrocellulose. Lanes 1–4 were stained with specific antisera to bFGF (1 : 1000): lane 1 = bovine bFGF standard (50 ng; 18 kDa); lane 2 = bovine aFGF standard (50 ng; 16 kDa); lane 3 = injured brain homogenate; lane 4 = intact brain homogenate; lane 5 = molecular weight standards; lanes 6–9 were stained with anti-bFGF sera pre-incubated with an excess of peptide immunogen (5 μg/μl whole sera); lane 6 = injured brain homogenate; lane 7 = intact brain homogenate; lane 8 = bovine aFGF standard; lane 9 = bovine bFGF standard. Three bands of bFGF immunoreactivity were found in rat brain homogenate (lanes 3 and 4; 18, 22, and 24 kDa; see text). Moreover, bFGF immunoreactivity was greater in homogenates from injured v. intact brain (lane 3 v. 4, respectively). Basic FGF immunoreactivity was abolished by pre-incubation of sera with peptide immunogen (lanes 6, 7, 9).

6, 7, 9; see legend). No difference in aFGF immunoreactivity in fractions from injured v. intact brain was seen on similar blots stained with anti-aFGF sera.

More recently, we have used heparin-affinity high performance liquid chromatography (HPLC) to further study relative changes in aFGF v. bFGF after brain injury (Finklestein *et al.*, 1990). Brain homogenates were loaded on to a heparin-TSK HPLC column, and retained proteins were eluted with a continuous gradient of 0.6–2.0 M NaCl, and assayed for mitogenic activity on Balb/c 3T3 cells, as above. These methods result in the clear separation of aFGF and bFGF in brain homogenate. Using these methods, we found a large increase in bFGF activity (c. 7-fold), and only a modest increase in aFGF activity (c. 1.7-fold) at one week after injury. Changes in bFGF bioactivity were paralleled by changes in bFGF immunoreactivity as seen on Western blots of column eluates (Finklestein *et al.*, 1990).

In other studies, we examined FGF levels following focal ischaemic injury (stroke) to the mature rat brain (Finklestein *et al.*, 1989b). Focal infarcts were made in the lateral cerebral cortex of mature Long–Evans rats by ligation of the carotid and middle cerebral arteries (Chen *et al.*, 1986). At various time points after stroke (0, 3, 7, 14, 21, 30 and 60 days), animals were sacrificed, and regions surrounding infarcts were dissected for FGF assay. FGF levels rose steadily to reach a peak of two to three times control values during the first 3 weeks after stroke, and remained elevated for at least 2 months following infarction. As was the case with mechanical brain injury, heparin-affinity HPLC showed that the increase in total FGF levels was due largely to increased levels of bFGF.

In immunohistochemical studies, we examined the localization of bFGF in the injured rat brain (Finklestein *et al.*, 1988). In the intact brain, bFGF immunoreactivity was localized primarily in neurons, especially in structures that are part of the brain's 'limbic system' (including hippocampus, hypothalamus, amygdala, and certain cortical regions). These results are especially intriguing, given the known capacity of these neurons for continued synaptic plasticity throughout life (Cotman and Nieto-Sampedro, 1984). In the injured brain, bFGF immunoreactivity was found at the borders of focal cortical wounds at 1 week after injury (Fig. 3(a)). This increase was due to the dense collection of bFGF-containing cells surrounding wounds (Fig. 3(b)). At high power (Fig. 3(c)), these cells have the appearance of 'reactive' micro- or astroglia. Thus, while bFGF is found primarily within neurons in the intact brain, glial cells appear to have the capacity to 'turn on' bFGF expression after injury.

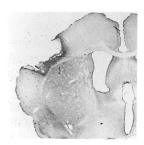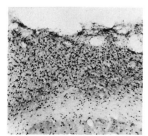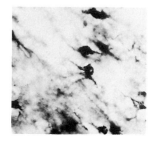

Figure 3. Immunohistochemical localization of bFGF in injured rat brain. Coronal sections (35 μm) of rat brain with focal suction lesions of the lateral cerebral cortex were immunostained with anti-bFGF sera at 1 week after injury. (Left) Increased bFGF immunoreactivity is seen at the borders of the focal brain wound. (Centre) At higher power (25×), bFGF immunoreactivity is seen to be localized to a dense collection of cells surrounding wounds. (Right) At highest power (40×), bFGF immunoreactivity is seen to be localized to stellate-shaped cells having the appearance of 'reactive' astroglia. (Part of figure reproduced with permission, from Finklestein *et al.*, 1988.)

In summary, our results show increased FGF levels following both mechanical and ischaemic injury (stroke) to the mature rat brain. This increase appears to be qualitatively similar but quantitatively greater after mechanical than similar-sized ischaemic wounds at 1 week after injury. Time course studies show a gradual increase in FGF levels during the first 3 weeks after stroke, persisting for at least 2 months. Bioassay and immunoassay techniques at selected time points show that the increased FGF levels after mechanical or ischaemic injury are due primarily to increased levels of bFGF. Immunohistochemical studies show that this increase is due to the dense accumulation of bFGF-containing cells surrounding wounds, most likely reactive glial cells. It is unclear to what extent bFGF remains localized in these cells or is released into the extracellular space. In previous studies (Finklestein et al., 1989a), we found increased 3T3-mitogenic activity in extracellular fluid preparations from the injured brain, suggesting increased bFGF release. However, aside from lysis of damaged cells, the mechanism of such release remains obscure, since the bFGF gene lacks a signal peptide sequence (Klagsbrun, 1990).

Because of its multipotential trophic effects, bFGF is likely to play an important role in wound healing in the CNS. By 1 week after injury, focal mechanical or ischaemic lesions of the mammalian CNS are surrounded by a dense network of proliferating capillaries and glial cells, as well as by early neural sprouting (Adams and Sidman, 1982; du Bois et al., 1985). As noted above, bFGF has potent gliotrophic, angiogenic, and neuronotrophic properties in tissue culture. Thus, the increased levels of bFGF that we observed in the first few weeks after injury may play an important role in the glial and capillary proliferation, as well as in the neural sprouting occurring during this time. The relative 'lag' in neural sprouting compared with other cellular reactions may be due to the necessity for retrograde transport of locally-expressed growth factor to distant neuronal cell bodies before axonal outgrowth can occur. Such sprouting, in particular, appears to contribute to functional recovery after injury (Azmitia et al., 1978; Cotman and Nieto-Sampedro, 1984).

Our results also shed light on possible differences in the role of aFGF v. bFGF in the mammalian brain. A priori, it is unclear why two such highly homologous factors are required in the CNS. Reported differences between these factors include different in vitro potencies, different potentiation by heparin, different susceptibilities to proteases, and perhaps different receptor sites on some cell types (Gospodarowicz et al., 1987; Klagsbrun, 1990). Our current findings suggest that these factors play different roles in the injured brain. At 1 week after injury, we found a large increase in bFGF levels, but only a modest increase in aFGF levels. Other investigators have reported larger increases in aFGF levels, occurring only during the first 2 days after injury (Nieto-Sampedro et al., 1988). Taken together, these findings suggest a different time course of expression, and consequently a different physiologic-al role for aFGF v. bFGF in the injured brain. Clearly, further studies are required to define the detailed time course of FGF expression after injury, to identify cell types expressing FGF receptors, and to determine the cellular and functional effects of FGF directly applied to the injured brain. Such studies may ultimately lead to the development of growth factors as pharmacological agents to accelerate wound healing after CNS injury.

ACKNOWLEDGEMENTS

Supported by NINDS NS10828, NIA AG08207, and a Grant-in-Aid from the American Heart Association (to S.F.), and by NCI CA37392 (to M.K.).

REFERENCES

Adams, R.D. and Sidman, R.L. (1982). *Introduction to Neuropathology*, McGraw-Hill, New York, pp. 172–174.

Adams, R.D. and Victor, M. (1985). *Principles of Neurology*, McGraw-Hill, New York.

Azmitia, E.C., Buchan, A.M. and Williams, J.H. (1978). Structural and functional restoration by collateral sprouting of hippocampal 5-HT axons. *Nature, 274*, 374–376.

Chen, S.T., Hsu, C.Y., Hogan, E.L., Maricq, H. and Balentine, J.D. (1986). A model of focal ischaemic stroke in the rat: reproducible extensive cortical infarction. *Stroke, 17*, 738–743.

Cotman, C.W. and Nieto-Sampedro, M. (1984). Cell biology of synaptic plasticity. *Science, 225*, 1267–1294.

Davidson, J.M. Klagsbrun, M., Hill, K.E., Buckley, A., Sullivan, R., Brewer, P.S. and Woodward, S.C. (1985). Accelerated wound repair, cell proliferation, and collagen accumulation are produced by a cartilage-derived growth factor. *J. Cell Biol., 100*, 1219–1227.

Du Bois, M., Bowman, P.D. and Goldstein, G.W. (1985). Cell proliferation after ischemic injury in gerbil brain. *Cell Tissue Res., 242*, 17–23.

Finklestein, S.P., Apostolides, P.J., Caday, C.G., Prosser, J., Philips, M.F. and Klagsbrun, M. (1988). Increased basic fibroblast growth factor (bFGF) immuno-reactivity at the site of focal brain wounds. *Brain Res., 460*, 253–259.

Finklestein, S.P., D'Amore, P.A., Caday, C.G. and Klagsbrun, M. (1989a). Angiogenic factors in brain. In: Ginsberg, M.D. and Dietrich, W.D. (Eds), *Cerebrovascular Diseases*, Raven Press, New York, pp. 425–429.

Finklestein, S.P., Caday, C.G., Kano, M., Foster, J., Hsu, C.Y., Liu, P.H., Moskowitz, M.A. and Klagsbrun, M. (1989b). FGF levels after stroke. *Soc. Neurosci. Abstr., 15*, 361.

Finklestein, S.P., Fanning, P.J., Caday, C.G., Powell, P.P., Foster, J., Clifford, E.M. and Klagsbrun, M. (1990). Increased levels of basic fibroblast growth factor (bFGF) following focal brain injury. *Res. Neurol. Neurosci.*, in press.

Folkman, J. and Klagsbrun, M. (1987). Angiogenic factors. *Science*, **235**, 442–447.

Gospodarowicz, D., Ferrara, N., Schweigerér, L. and Neufeld, G. (1987). Structural characterization and biological functions of fibroblast growth factor. *Endocrine Rev.*, **8**, 95–114.

Klagsbrun, M. (1990). The fibroblast growth factor family: Structural and biological properties. *Prog. Growth Factor Res.*, in press.

Klagsbrun, M. and Shing, Y. (1985). Heparin affinity of anionic and cationic capillary endothelial cell growth factors: Analysis of hypothalamus-derived growth factors and fibroblast growth factors. *Proc. Natl Acad. Sci. USA*, **82**, 805–809.

Moscatelli, D., Joseph-Silverstein, J., Manejias, R. and Rifkin, D.B. (1987). M_r 25,000 heparin-binding protein from guinea pig brain is a high molecular weight form of basic fibroblast growth factor. *Proc. Natl Acad. Sci. USA*, **84**, 5778–5782.

Nieto-Sampedro, M., Lim, R., Hicklin, D.J. and Cotman, C.W. (1988). Early release of glia maturation factor and acidic fibroblast growth factor after rat brain injury. *Neurosci. Lett.*, **86**, 361–365.

Pettman, B., Weibel, M., Sensenbrenner, M. and Labourdette, G. (1985). Purification of two astroglial growth factors from bovine brain. *FEBS Lett.*, **189**, 102–108.

Wadzinski, M.G., Folkman, J., Sasse, J., Devey, K., Ingber, D. and Klagsbrun, M. (1987). Heparin-binding angiogenesis factors: Detection by immunological methods. *Clin. Physiol. Biochem.*, **5**, 200–209.

Walicke, P.A. (1988). Basic and acidic fibroblast growth factors have trophic effects on neurons from multiple CNS regions. *J. Neurosci.*, **8**, 2618–2627.

Wound Healing
Edited by H. Janssen, R. Rooman and J.I.S. Robertson
© 1991 Wrightson Biomedical Publishing Ltd

6

Synergistic Interaction of Transmembrane Signalling Pathways in Growth Factor Action

KLAUS SEUWEN and JACQUES POUYSSÉGUR

Biochemical Research Centre, CNRS, University of Nice-Sophia Antipolis, Nice, France

Growth factors are agents that promote, alone or in combination, the multiplication of well nourished cells. Much of our current knowledge concerning their action has been obtained through studies of cells cultivated *in vitro*, especially rodent fibroblasts, that can be easily established as stable cell lines. The development of serum-free culture media has greatly facilitated the identification of mitogenic molecules and has allowed study of diverse aspects of their action under defined conditions. In recent years, many molecules that had been formerly known to mediate other biological responses, like neurotransmitters, neurohormones and vasoactive agents have been found to stimulate cell proliferation. In most experimental systems, these agents do not show spectacular effects if applied alone, but synergize with other growth factors to produce a strong proliferative response. How do growth factors act and interact? What do we know about the biochemical events transducing cell proliferation signals?

GROWTH FACTOR RECEPTORS AND INTRACELLULAR MESSENGERS

Growth factors seem to use at least two different strategies for transmembrane signal transduction. The polypeptides platelet-derived growth factor (PDGF), epidermal growth factor (EGF), fibroblast growth factor (FGF), and colony stimulating factor-1 (CSF-1), act through receptors containing an intrinsic ligand-activated tyrosine kinase (Yarden and Ullrich, 1988). The primary structures of these receptors are known today and interestingly there are no indications so far for receptors subtypes with different functions. For a long time the intracellular substrates of the tyrosine kinases relevant for growth control have remained elusive, but recently it was discovered that the raf-1 protein can be directly phosphorylated by the PDGF receptor (Morrison *et al.*, 1989). The raf-1 protein is a serine kinase implicated in growth control and the phosphorylation on tyrosine activates the kinase. These results favour the hypothesis that the tyrosine kinase receptors are the first of a cascade of kinases.

On the other hand, the growth promoting agents thrombin, bombesin, bradykinin, vasopressin and serotonin seem to act through different mechanisms. These molecules have in common the ability to activate phosphoinositide (PI) breakdown, and/or inhibit adenylate cyclase (AC). Recent evidence suggests that activation of PI specific phospholipase C (PLC) and inhibition of AC are mediated by different receptor subtypes coupling differentially to regulatory G proteins, which are supposed to control PLC or AC activity (Lefkowitz and Caron, 1988; Ashkenazi *et al.*, 1989). Hormone receptors interacting with these regulatory proteins seemingly have a common structure, resembling the rhodopsin 'prototype': they are large monomeric molecules of about 50 kDa thought to integrate into the plasma membrane through seven membrane spanning α-helices. The primary structures of the three serotonin receptors cloned so far (5-HT$_{1c}$, 5-HT$_2$, 5-HT$_{1a}$) fit exactly into this family (Julius *et al.*, 1988; Pritchett *et al.*, 1988; Fargin *et al.*, 1989). The sequence of receptors of the other agents cited, however, is still unknown.

It is generally assumed that the mitogenic effect of this family of growth factors is due to their stimulatory effect on PI turnover. In fact, the activation of this signalling pathway can explain most of the early events generally observed after addition of growth factors to quiescent cells. We have to keep in mind, however, that these events are also elicited by the growth factors of the tyrosine kinase class, which do not or only weakly activate PI turnover in untransformed cells. Therefore, parallel pathways seem to exist for growth factor action. Taking the example of the CCL39 hamster lung fibroblast cell line, we will in the following discuss some aspects of growth factor signal transduction, focusing especially on the role of agents activating G protein coupled receptors and their synergistic interaction with 'tyrosine kinase growth factors'.

CCL39 CELLS AS A MODEL SYSTEM TO STUDY GROWTH CONTROL

CCL39 is a diploid cell line established from Chinese hamster lung fibroblasts that has been used for 10 years in this laboratory as a model to study growth

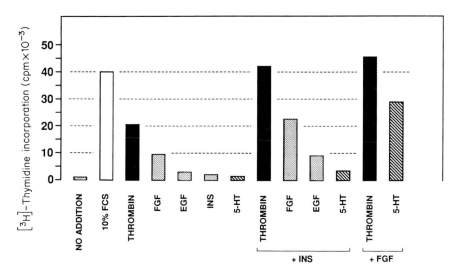

Figure 1. Stimulation of DNA synthesis by different growth factors in CCL39 cells. Confluent cell monolayers were rendered quiescent by a 24 h incubation in serum-free medium. The cells were then stimulated with the growth factors indicated in the presence of [³H]thymidine. FCS = fetal calf serum. After 24 h, radioactivity incorporated into trichloroacetic acid precipitable material was counted. The growth factors were used in the following concentrations: thrombin, 10 nM; FGF, 50 ng/ml; EGF, 50 ng/ml; INS, 5 µg/ml; 5-HT, 10 µM.

control and signal transduction. These cells can be arrested in the G0/G1 phase of the cell cycle by incubation in serum-free medium and remain viable in the presence of insulin (INS) and transferrin for several days in their quiescent state. A limited set of hormones and growth factors including α-thrombin (THR), serotonin (5-HT), EGF, FGF and insulin-like growth factor 1 (IGF-1) is capable of inducing DNA synthesis (Fig. 1) and continuous cell proliferation in serum-free medium (Pérez-Rodriguez *et al.*, 1981; Magnaldo *et al.*, 1986; L'Allemain and Pouysségur, 1986).

THROMBIN AS A GROWTH FACTOR

α-Thrombin (THR) is the most potent mitogen for these cells uncovered so far. THR alone is able to initiate DNA synthesis in 30–40% of a quiescent cell population. This is rather exceptional, as growth factors usually exhibit relatively weak effects on normal cells if applied alone. In order to achieve a similar stimulation of growth, two or three growth factors acting in synergy usually have to be applied. Thrombin strongly activates PI turnover and inhibits AC and we therefore class it in the family of growth factors acting through G protein coupled receptors (Pouysségur *et al.*, 1988). Direct proof that G proteins are involved in thrombin's action came from experiments where the effect of Pertussis toxin (PTX) on cell proliferation induced by different growth factors was studied. This bacterial toxin was orginally discovered to enhance insulin secretion in pancreatic islets, hence its second name 'islet activating protein' (Ui, 1984). The effect on islets turned out to be correlated with the toxin-induced ADP-ribosylation of 'G_i', the inhibitory G protein of AC, leading to its functional uncoupling from the cyclase. But PTX also affected PLC activation in some cells and it was assumed that the postulated G protein regulating PI breakdown was in these instances a PTX substrate (Cockcroft, 1987). In CCL39 cells, PTX inhibited thrombin induced PLC activation by about 50% (Paris and Pouysségur, 1986) and it was tempting to check whether the substance interferred with thrombin induced DNA synthesis. In fact, the mitogenic potential of thrombin was strongly antagonized by PTX treatment, whereas the actions of insulin, EGF and FGF remained unaffected (Chambard *et al.*, 1987). These data clearly demonstrated the physiological importance of G proteins in growth factor action. The fact that the growth factors activating receptor tyrosine kinases are not antagonized by PTX elegantly confirmed the concept of the two classes of receptors using distinct mechanisms of signal transduction. Similar results were independently reported by Letterio *et al.* (1986) who compared the action of Bombesin (PTX-sensitive) and PDGF (PTX-insensitive) in Swiss 3T3 cells.

SEROTONIN STIMULATES DNA SYNTHESIS THROUGH A RECEPTOR NEGATIVELY COUPLED TO AC

To most of us it seemed obvious that the PTX-sensitive step in the action of growth factors like thrombin and bombesin was the activation of PI breakdown. However, experiments with serotonin carried out with our cell system confronted us for the first time with results showing that PLC activation and stimulation of DNA synthesis could be dissociated.

Serotonin is not a mitogen on its own in CCL39 cells; but if applied together with FGF, it strongly stimulates DNA synthesis (Fig. 1) and this effect can be completely blocked by PTX (Seuwen *et al.*, 1988). CCL39 cells express two serotonin receptors: 5-HT_2, activating ·PLC, and 5-HT_{1b}, inhibiting AC. To our surprise, we found that the action of serotonin as a growth factor depended on the activation of the latter receptor, whereas activation of PI breakdown by 5-HT_2 receptors had no measurable effect (Seuwen *et al.*, 1988; Seuwen and Pouysségur, 1990). These results explained the PTX-effect on serotonin induced DNA synthesis in a straightforward manner. One or more G_i proteins, classical substrates of PTX, seemed to be involved.

α_2-ADRENERGIC AGONISTS AS GROWTH FACTORS

In order to verify that receptors negatively coupled to AC can stimulate DNA synthesis, we decided to express in CCL39 cells α_2-adrenergic receptors, recently cloned by Kobilka and coworkers (1987). These receptors are known to regulate a variety of physiological functions exhibiting the same effector coupling specificity as 5-HT_{1b} receptors. Indeed we found that the α_2-agonists epinephrine and clonidine behaved like serotonin in the transfected cells: they inhibited AC and stimulated DNA synthesis in synergy with FGF and this effect was completely PTX-sensitive (Fig. 2; Seuwen et al., 1990a). Moreover, serotonin and epinephrine action in these cells is not additive, suggesting a common signal transduction pathway.

WHAT IS THE ROLE OF cAMP IN THE CONTROL OF CELL PROLIFERATION?

Can a decrease in intracellular cAMP levels brought about by serotonin or epinephrine explain the stimulation of cell growth? Depending on the cell system studies, cAMP can either have stimulatory or inhibitory effects. In Swiss 3T3 cells (Rozengurt et al., 1981) as well as in various epithelial cells (Dumont et al., 1989). increased levels of cAMP promote proliferation, whereas the contrary is true for most other cells (Pastan et al., 1975) including CCL39 fibroblasts. Here, hormones stimulating AC, like prostaglandin E_1 (PGE_1), strongly inhibit proliferation independently of the growth factor used to stimulate it (Magnaldo et al., 1989). Conversely, any agent inhibiting cAMP production might therefore increase proliferation. Unfortunately, it is difficult to test this hypothesis because there is no way to lower cAMP levels in intact cells without using hormones activating G_i and the possibility exists that other, so far unknown, messenger systems controlled by G_i proteins are at the origin of the growth response. Interestingly, in platelets as well as in pancreatic islet cells, the α_2 agonist epinephrine does not seem to act through a decrease in cAMP (Haslam et al., 1978; Ullrich and Wollheim, 1984).

Several different biochemical systems in addition to PLC and AC are known or are supposed to be regulated by G proteins. Ionic channels and other phospholipases as well as tyrosine kinases, have received attention recently and it will be important to evaluate these different possibilities.

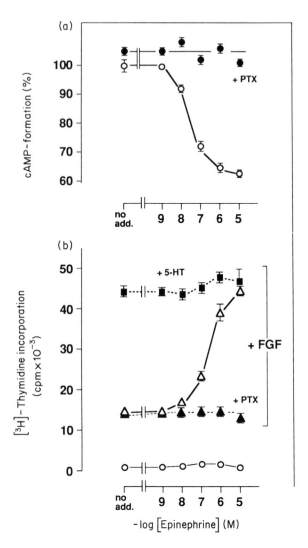

Figure 2. Effect of epinephrine on adenylate cyclase activity (a) and reinitiation of DNA synthesis (b) in CCL39 cells expressing α_2-adrenergic receptors. DNA synthesis experiments were carried out as described in Fig. 1, AC measurements as described previously (Magnaldo *et al.*, 1988; Seuwen *et al.*, 1988). ●, ○ = epinephrine added alone; △, ▲ = epinephrine added in the presence of FGF (50 ng/ml); ●, ▲ = cells pretreated for 4 h with PTX (150 ng/ml); ■ = epinephrine added in the presence of FGF (50 ng/ml and 5-HT 10 µM).

SIMILARITIES BETWEEN THROMBIN AND SEROTONIN ACTION

Like serotonin, thrombin activates PLC and inhibits AC. There are two major differences, however. The first and more important difference is that thrombin activates PI turnover much more strongly then serotonin does (Seuwen and Pouysségur, 1990). The second point is that this activation requires much higher thrombin concentrations than the inhibition of AC (Paris and Pouysségur, 1986; Magnaldo et al., 1988). In the case of serotonin, both biochemical events can be observed over roughly the same concentration range of agonist (Seuwen et al., 1988). Interestingly, at low thrombin concentrations (<0.1 nM), no or only a very weak stimulation of PLC activity and no mitogenic effect is detectable, but the same doses fully inhibit AC and elicit a strong DNA synthesis response in synergy with FGF (Paris et al., 1988; Magnaldo et al., 1988; Seuwen et al., 1989). Therefore, thrombin at low concentrations acts much like serotonin. Only at high concentrations (typically 10 nM), it becomes a powerful mitogen on its own. It is noteworthy, too, that thrombin and serotonin do not produce additive or synergistic effects in the DNA synthesis assay, which is compatible with the notion that thrombin is capable of producing the same signal serotonin is generating.

STRONG ACTIVATION OF PLC IS NOT A SUFFICIENT MITOGENIC SIGNAL

Thrombin is the strongest pure PLC agonist in CCL39 cells. In order to test the hypothesis that this pathway mediates the biological effects of the growth factor, we needed a possibility to activate it to a similar degree in the absence of thrombin. The recent molecular cloning of several receptors specifically coupled to PLC made this approach possible. As for the α_2-adrenergic receptor, we used DNA transfection to express human muscarinic M1 acetylcholine receptors (Peralta et al., 1987) and 5-HT$_{1c}$ receptors (Julius et al., 1988) in CCL39 cells. We obtained functional expression of both receptors and using carbachol (Fig. 3) or serotonin, respectively, we could now stimulate PI turnover to the same extent and even stronger than with thrombin. However, we could not observe significant stimulation of DNA synthesis under these conditions (Fig. 3). The non-effect of carbachol and serotonin on cell proliferation compared with thrombin can apparently not be attributed to a qualitatively or quantitatively different PLC response, as we failed so far to detect significant differences in the production of IP$_2$ and IP$_3$ inside cells as well as Ca^{2+} release from intracellular stores (Suewen et al., 1990b).

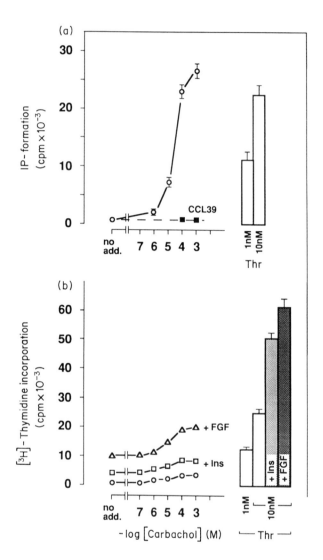

Figure 3. Effect of carbachol on PI turnover (a) and DNA synthesis (b) in CCL39 cells expressing muscarinic M1 acetylcholine receptors. Comparison with thrombin. Release of IPs was measured as described previously (Seuwen *et al.*, 1988), DNA synthesis experiments as described in Fig. 1. ○ = carbachol added alone; △ = carbachol added in the presence of FGF (50 ng/ml); □ = carbachol added in the presence of INS (5 μg/ml); ■ = carbachol does not activate PI turnover in untransfected CCL39 cells.

These data show that even a strong activation of PI turnover cannot be considered sufficient to induce a proliferative response in CCL39 cells. Again, only in synergy with FGF can an appreciable response be observed. In the case of carbachol, this effect remains rather weak (Fig. 3), whereas thrombin elicits the same strong synergistic response with insulin and FGF as in untransfected CCL39 cells.

Our data suggest that the known G protein-mediated biochemical effects elicited by thrombin, activation of PLC and inhibition of AC, both mimicked by serotonin in the 5-HT$_{1c}$ receptor transfected CCL39 cells, are not sufficient to explain its mitogenicity. Therefore, thrombin probably does use yet other transmembrane signalling mechanisms acting in synergy with the above mentioned pathways. At present, we cannot exclude the possibility that it activates a receptor tyrosine kinase or a G protein-activated kinase.

CONCLUSIONS

We have shown that expression of G protein coupled receptors (stimulating PLC or inhibiting AC) did not generate cells that responded to the appropriate agonist alone in the DNA synthesis assay. In both cases the action depended on the parallel activation of a receptor of the tyrosine kinase class (FGF), which is able to elicit a significant growth response on its own (Fig. 1). Surprisingly, agents acting through G$_i$ coupled receptors evoked stronger synergistic responses with FGF than agents activating the PLC pathway.

Our data indicate that growth factors of the tyrosine kinase class are 'master growth factors' determining to what degree cells will respond to agents acting through G protein coupled receptors. The relative importance of the tyrosine kinase pathway(s) is reflected by the fact that a large number of virus encoded oncogenes exist that code for aberrant receptors of this kind, whereas no naturally occurring virus has so far been found to carry a receptor with seven potential transmembrane domains. In fact, overexpression of normal receptors of the tyrosine kinase class in CCL39 fibroblasts yields cells that respond very well to the appropriate ligand alone, up to showing a ligand dependent transformed phenotype (L'Allemain *et al.*, 1989; Hartmann *et al.*, 1990). Although transfection of the angiotensin receptor and the 5-HT$_{1c}$ receptor has been reported to deregulate cell growth, the two ligands did not act as strong mitogens in the transfected cells and tumour formation in nude mice seems to depend on additional lesions, as recovered tumour cells proved to be largely growth factor independent *in vitro* and showed a transformed phenotype in the absence of angiotensin or serotonin, respectively (Jackson *et al.*, 1988; Julius *et al.*, 1989). These growth deregulating lesions could well be located somewhere on the tyrosine kinase pathway. Our data predict that constitutive activation of this pathway, for instance by a mutated ligand independent receptor, should render cells responsive to hormones acting through G protein coupled receptors.

Thrombin is an exceptionally potent mitogen in CCL39 cells that acts through several parallel pathways including PLC activation, AC inhibition and at least one further unknown mechanism which seems functionally equivalent to the activation of a receptor tyrosine kinase. It will be an important issue of future work to understand in more detail how these pathways converge to produce a strong proliferative response.

ACKNOWLEDGEMENTS

We thank Martine Valetti for expert secretarial work. This work was supported by grants from the Centre National de la Recherche Scientifique (UPR 7300), the Institut National de la Santé et de la Recherche Médicale, the Fondation pour la Recherche Médicale and the Association pour la Recherche contre le Cancer.

REFERENCES

Ashkenazi, A., Peralta, E.G., Winslow, J.W., Ramachandran, J. and Capon, J. (1989). Functionally distinct G proteins selectively couple different receptors to PI hydrolysis in the same cells. *Cell*, **56**, 487–493.

Chambard, J.C., Paris, S., L'Allemain, G. and Pouysségur, J. (1987). Two growth factors signalling pathways in fibroblasts distinguished by pertussis toxin. *Nature*, **326**, 800–803.

Cockcroft, S. (1987). Polyphosphoinositide phosphodiesterase regulatory by a novel guanine nucleotide binding protein Gp. *Trends Biochem, Sci.*, **12**, 75–78.

Dumont, J.E., Jauniaux, J.C. and Roger, P.P. (1989). The cAMP mediated stimulation of cell proliferation. *Trends Biochem. Sci.*, **14**, 67–71.

Fargin, A., Raymond, J.R., Lohse, M.J., Kobilka, B.K., Caron, M.G. and Lefkowitz, R.J. (1989). The genomic clone G-21 which resembles a β-adrenergic receptor sequence encodes the 5-HT$_{1A}$ receptor. *Nature*, **335**, 358–360.

Hartmann, T., Seuwen, K., Roussel, M.F., Sherr, C.J. and Pouysségur, J. (1990). Functional expression of the human receptor for colony-stimulating factor 1 (CSF-1) in hamster fibroblasts stimulates Na$^+$/H$^+$ exchange and DNA-synthesis in the absence of phosphoinositide breakdown. *Growth Factors*, **2**, 289–300.

Haslam, R.J., Davidson, M.M.L. and Desjardins, S.V. (1978). Inhibition of adenylate cyclase by adenosine analogues in preparations of broken and intact human platelets. Evidence for the unidirectional control of platelet function by cyclic AMP. *Biochem. J.*, **176**, 83–95.

Jackson, T.R., Blair, L.A.C., Marshall, J., Goedert, M. and Hanley, M.R. (1988). The mas oncogene encodes an angiotensin receptor. *Nature*, **335**, 437–440.

Julius, D., McDermott, A.B., Axel, R. and Jessel, T.M. (1988). Molecular characterization of functional cDNA encoding the serotonin 1c receptor. *Science*, **241**, 558–564.

Julius, D., Livelli, T.J., Jessell, T.M. and Axel, R. (1989). Ectopic expression of the serotonin 1c receptor and the triggering of malignant transformation. *Science*, **244**, 1057–1062.

Kobilka, B.K., Frielle, T., Collins, S., Yang-Freng, T., Kobilka, T.S., Francke, U., Lefkowitz, R.J. and Caron, M.G. (1987). An intronless gene encoding a potential member of the family of receptors coupled to guanine nucleotide regulatory proteins. *Nature*, **329**, 75–79.

L'Allemain, G. and Pouysségur, J. (1986). EGF and insulin action in fibroblasts: evidence that phosphoinositide hydrolysis is not an essential mitogenic signalling pathway. *FEBS Lett.*, **197**, 344–348.

L'Allemain, G., Seuwen, K., Velu, T. and Pouysségur, J. (1989). Signal transduction in hamster fibroblasts overexpressing the human EGF receptor. *Growth Factors*, **1**, 311–321.

Lefkowitz, R.J. and Caron, M.G. (1988). Adrenergic receptors. Models for the study of receptors coupled to guanine nucleotide regulatory proteins. *J. Biol. Chem.*, **263**, 4993–4996.

Letterio, J.J., Coughlin, S.R. and Williams, L.T. (1986). Pertussis toxin-sensitive pathway in the stimulation of c-myc expression and DNA synthesis by bombesin. *Science*, **234**, 1117–1119.

Magnaldo, I., L'Allemain, G., Chambard, J.C., Moenner, M., Barritault, D. and Pouysségur, J. (1986). The mitogenic-signalling pathway of FGF is not mediated through polyphosphoinositide hydrolysis and protein kinase C activation in hamster fibroblasts. *J. Biol. Chem.*, **261**, 16916–16922.

Magnaldo, I., Pouysségur, J. and Paris, S. (1988). Thrombin exerts a dual effect on stimulated adenylate cyclase in hamster fibroblasts: an inhibition via a GTP-binding protein and a potentiation via activation of protein kinase C. *Biochem. J.*, **253**, 711–719.

Magnaldo, I., Pouysségur, J. and Paris, S. (1989). Cyclic AMP inhibits mitogen-induced DNA synthesis in hamster fibroblasts regardless of the signalling pathway involved. *FEBS Lett.*, **245**, 65–69.

Morrison, D.K., Kaplan, D.R., Escobedo, J.A., Rapp, U.R., Roberts, T.M. and Williams, L.T. (1989). Direct activation of the serine/threonine kinase activity of Raf-1 through tyrosine phosphorylation by the PDGF β-receptor. *Cell*, **58**, 649–657.

Paris, S. and Pouysségur, J. (1986). Pertussis toxin inhibits thrombin-induced activation of phosphoinositide hydrolysis and Na$^+$/H$^+$ exchange in hamster fibroblasts. *EMBO J.*, **5**, 55–60.

Paris, S., Chambard, J.C. and Pouysségur, J. (1988). Tyrosine kinase-activating growth factors potentiate thrombin- and A1F^{4-} induced phosphoinositide breakdown in hamster fibroblasts: evidence for positive cross-talk between the two mitogenic signalling. *J. Biol. Chem.*, **263**, 12893–12900.

Pastan, I.H., Johnson, G.S. and Anderson, W.B. (1975). Role of cyclic nucleotides in growth control. *Ann. Rev. Biochem.*, **44**, 491–522.

Peralta, E.G., Ashkenazi, A., Winslow, A., Smith, D.H., Ramachandran, J. and Capon, D.J. (1987). Distinct primary structure, ligand-binding properties and tissue-specific expression of four human muscarinic acetylcholine receptors. *EMBO J.*, **6**, 3923–3929.

Pérez-Rodriguez, R., Franchi, A. and Pouysségur, J. (1981). Growth factor requirements of chinese hamster lung fibroblasts in serum free media: high mitogenic action of thrombin. *Cell Biol. Int. Rep.*, **5**, 347–357.

Pouysségur, J., Chambard, J.C. L'Allemain, G., Magnaldo, I and Seuwen, K. (1988). Transmembrane signalling pathways initiating cell growth in fibroblasts. *Phil. Trans. R. Soc. Lond.*, **B320**, 427–436.

Pritchett, D.B., Bach, A.W.J., Wozny, M., Taleb, O., Dal Toso, R., Shih, J.C. and Seeburg, P.H. (1988). Structure and functional expression of cloned rat serotonin 5-HT$_2$ receptor. *EMBO J.*, **7**, 4135–4140.

Rozengurt, E., Legg, A., Strang, G. and Courtenay-Luck, N. (1981). Cyclic AMP: a mitogenic signal for Swiss 3T3 cells. *Proc. Natl Acad. Sci. USA*, **78**, 4392–4396.

Seuwen, K. and Pouysségur, J. (1990). Serotonin as a growth factor. *Biochem. Pharmacol.*, **39**, 985–990.

Seuwen, K., Magnaldo, I. and Pouysségur, J. (1988). Serotonin stimulates DNA synthesis in fibroblasts acting through 5-HT$_{1B}$ receptors coupled to a G$_I$ protein. *Nature*, **335**, 254–256.

Seuwen, K., Chambard, J.C., L'Allemain, G., Magnaldo, I., Paris, S. and Pouysségur, J. (1989). Thrombin as a growth factor: mechanism of signal transduction. In: Meyer, P. and Marche, P. (Eds), *Blood, Cell and Arteries in Hypertension and Atherosclerosis*, Raven Press, New York, pp. 217–232.

Seuwen, K., Magnaldo, I., Kobilka, B.K., Caron, M.G., Regan, J.W., Lefkowitz, R.J. and Pouysségur, J. (1990a). α_2-Adrenergic agonists stimulate DNA synthesis in chinese hamster lung fibroblasts trasfected with human α_2-adrenergic receptor gene. *Cell Regulation*, **1**, 445–451.

Seuwen, K., Kahan, C., Hartmann, T., Capon, D. and Pousségur, J. (1990b). Strong and persistent activation of inositol lipid breakdown induces early mitogenic events but not G0 to S-phase progression in hamster fibroblasts. Comparison of thrombin and carbachol action in cells expressing m1 muscarinic acetylcholine receptors. *J. Biol, Chem.*, in press.

Ui, M. (1984). Islet-activating protein, pertussis toxin: a probe for functions of the inhibitory guanine nucleotide regulatory component of adenylate cyclase. *Trends Pharmacol. Sci.*, **5**, 277–279.

Ullrich, S. and Wollheim, C.B. (1984). Islet cyclic AMP levels are not lowered during α_2-adrenergic inhibition of insulin-release. *J. Biol. Chem.*, **259**, 4111–4115.

Yarden, Y. and Ullrich, A. (1988). Growth factor receptor tyrosine kinases. *Ann. Rev. Biochem.*, **57**, 443–470.

Wound Healing
Edited by H. Janssen, R. Rooman and J.I.S. Robertson
© 1991 Wrightson Biomedical Publishing Ltd

7

Regulation of Connective Tissue Turnover by Metalloproteinase Inhibitors

MICHAEL J. BANDA[1], ERIC W. HOWARD[1], G. SCOTT HERRON[2], GERARD APODACA[3,4] and GILLIAN MURPHY[5]

[1]Laboratory of Radiobiology and Environmental Health and Departments of [2]Dermatology, [3]Anatomy and [4]Pathology, University of California, San Francisco, California, USA, and [5]Strangeways Research Laboratory, Cambridge, UK

Debridement and connective tissue remodelling are as essential to successful wound healing as is the replacement of cellular tissue at the wound site. The latter process is probably the result of the coordinated action of several growth factors. The details of the coordination and the identity of the growth factors are not fully understood. However, the direct effect of a growth factor or factors cannot account for the regulated turnover of connective tissue that occurs during wound healing in general and during angiogenesis in particular. During the debridement phase of wound healing it is likely that the damaged components of the extracellular matrix are degraded by several robust serine proteinases derived from inflammatory neutrophils and macrophages, which are the first cells to infiltrate the wound site. Subsequently, proteinases of mesenchymal and endothelial origin are active during the infiltration of fibroblasts and the process of angiogenesis, respectively. These proteinases are members of a structurally related family of matrix metalloproteinases that includes interstitial collagenases, stromelysin, and the gelatinases or type IV collagenases.

The growth of new blood vessels during angiogenesis is associated with three distinct responses by the microvascular endothelium (Folkman, 1984). Capillary endothelial cells, which ultimately form the growth tip of a new capillary sprout, must first degrade and breach the basement membrane surrounding intact capillaries. They must then migrate through the extracellular matrix toward the source of the angiogenic stimulus. Proliferation of cells behind the migrating front and formation of a vascular lumen are major events associated with the final phase (Ausprunk and Folkman, 1977; Burger et al., 1983). The induction and arrest of capillary endothelial cell migration during neovascularization and angiogenesis require precise regulation of metalloproteinase activity.

The regulation of mammalian matrix-degrading metalloproteinases by endogenous protein inhibitors of metalloproteinases has generally been considered to be the result of the action of the tissue inhibitor of metalloproteinases (TIMP, M_r 30 000). Although TIMP can inhibit most secreted mammalian metalloproteinases, detailed studies of the kinetics of TIMP-metalloproteinase interaction have been limited to very few metalloproteinases, most notably interstitial collagenase (Cawston et al., 1983; Welgus et al., 1985). Whether TIMP is a biologically important inhibitor of all metalloproteinases remains to be determined. Studies in vitro have shown that TIMP can regulate the invasiveness of tumour cells (Mignatti et al., 1986) as well as chondrocytes and microvascular endothelial cells (Gavrilovic et al., 1987). Antisense TIMP RNA has a similar effect on Swiss 3T3 cells (Khokha et al., 1989). Although the extent to which TIMP-mediated inhibition is biologically significant is not known, it is generally accepted that TIMP is an important secreted protein inhibitor of metalloproteinases, particularly of interstitial collagenase. It is certainly the best characterized inhibitor of its type, and its entire amino acid sequence has been determined (Docherty et al., 1985).

There have been reports of other inhibitors of metalloproteinases that appear to be distinct from TIMP. Such inhibitors have been detected in chick embryonic cartilage (Yasui et al., 1981), human polymorphonuclear leukocytes (Macartney and Tschesche, 1983), and bovine cartilage (Bunning et al., 1984; Murray et al., 1986). All of these inhibitors have a lower molecular weight than human TIMP. It is not clear in all cases how the inhibitors are related to TIMP.

STUDIES WITH RABBIT ENDOTHELIAL CELLS

Because microvascular endothelial cells must migrate through the extracellular matrix during angiogenesis, we examined the expression of interstitial collagenase and stromelysin by rabbit brain capillary endothelial cells (RBCE) (Herron et al., 1986a). After stimulation by 12-O-tetradecanoylphorbol-13-acetate (TPA), RBCE expressed very little collagenase or stromelysin activity on a per cell basis when compared with rabbit synovial fibroblasts (RSF) (Table 1). Densitometric analysis of SDS–polyacrylamide gels showed no significant difference in the amount of collagenase and stromelysin protein secreted by the two cell types (Herron et al., 1986a). To determine if an endogenous inhibitor could be regulating these proteinase activities, an antibody to TIMP was used to absorb any TIMP present in the medium conditioned by RBCE. The removal of TIMP restored almost all of

Table 1. Collagenase and stromelysin activities in conditioned medium of TPA-treated RBCE and RSF[a].

Time after TPA addition (h)	Collagenase (units/10^5 cells)		Stromelysin (units/10^5 cells)	
	RBCE	RSF	RBCE	RSF
8	0	0	0	0
15	0	0.1	0.1	ND[b]
24	0	3.4	0.2	3.5
31	0.05	3.8	ND	ND
48	0.10	4.1	0.7	21.0

[a]RBCE and RSF were treated with 80 nM TPA in serum-free Dulbecco's modified Eagle's medium. At the indicated times, conditioned medium was removed and assayed for activatable metalloproteinases. (Reproduced with permission, from Herron et al. (1986b), © The American Society for Biochemistry and Molecular Biology, Inc.)
[b]ND, not determined.

the activity of collagenase and stromelysin (Table 2). This experiment does not demonstrate that all of the metalloproteinase activity was restored by the removal of TIMP, only that of collagenase and stromelysin. Gelatin zymography of the conditioned medium showed that the dominant metalloproteinase activities were associated with the gelatinases at M_r 68 000 and M_r 92 000, and the effect of TIMP removal on those proteinases was not addressed.

Because removal of TIMP from the RBCE-conditioned medium resulted in an increase in the activity of some metalloproteinases, the RBCE-conditioned medium was analysed by reverse-gelatin zymography (Herron et al., 1986b). Figure 1 shows the presence of TIMP as well as verification of its identity by immunoprecipitation with anti-TIMP antibody. In addition, two other inhibitors of metalloproteinases (IMPs) lower in molecular size than TIMP were detected in the medium at M_r 26 000 (IMP-1) and M_r 21 000 (IMP-2). These data suggest that, in addition to TIMP, at least two other inhibitory proteins are secreted by rabbit endothelial cells.

EXPRESSION OF IMPS BY HUMAN CELLS

Because malignant gliomas rarely metastasize, we examined the medium conditioned by fetal human astrocytes and cells from five glioma cell lines for expression of metalloproteinases and their inhibitors. The conditioned

Table 2. Collagenase and stromelysin activities in
conditioned medium of TPA-treated RBCE before and
after removal of TIMP[a].

Time after TPA addition (h)	Collagenase (units/10^5 cells)		Stromelysin (units/10^5 cells)	
	TIMP present	TIMP removed	TIMP present	TIMP removed
Control[b]	0	0	0	0
24	0	0	0.8	2.0
48	0	2.5	2.8	7.6
56	0.7	4.2	4.0	11.2

[a]RBCE were treated and assayed as described in Table 1. TIMP
was removed by incubation of conditioned medium with
anti-TIMP-affinity resin.
[b]Control cells were incubated for 56 h without TPA.

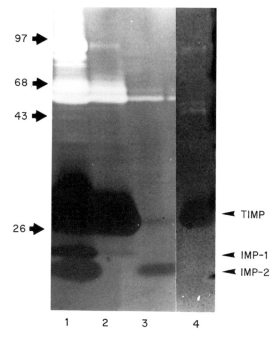

Figure 1. Characterization of inhibitors from RBCE by SDS-gelatin zymography.
Conditioned medium from RBCE treated with 80 nM TPA (lane 1) was separated on
Sephacryl S-200, and selected fractions containing inhibitor activity were analysed by
reverse gelatin zymography (lanes 2 and 3). Lane 4 shows the bound and eluted
protein incubated with anti-TIMP-affinity resin. Molecular weight markers ($M_r \times 10^{-3}$) are shown at the left. (Reproduced with permission, from Herron *et al.* (1986a),
© The American Society for Biochemistry and Molecular Biology, Inc.)

medium from these cells did not degrade azocoll in suspension, but several proteolytic activities, inhibitable by 1,10-phenanthroline, were detected by gelatin zymography. After treatment with TPA, the secretion of the M_r 92 000, 57 000, and 52 000 proteinases was induced or enhanced in all of the cells. The M_r 92 000 and 65 000 proteinases bound specifically to a gelatin affinity column. When purified by preparative gel electrophoresis, the M_r 65 000 proteinase was found to degrade type IV procollagen. The M_r 57 000 and 52 000 species were precipitated by anti-collagenase IgG. TIMP was detected in the conditioned medium of all the cells by analysis with reverse zymography and immunoprecipitation of [^{35}S]methionine-labelled proteins with anti-TIMP IgG (Fig. 2). In addition to TIMP, the glioma cells, but not the fetal astrocytes, also secreted various amounts of the two IMPs seen in RBCE-conditioned medium (IMP-1 at M_r 26 000 and IMP-2 at M_r 21 000), and a third IMP (IMP-3), not previously identified, at M_r 18 000. Because normal adult astrocyte cell lines were not available, it was impossible to determine whether the expression of IMPs is a normal characteristic of adult cells or the result of transformation to a glioma. The stimulation by TPA affected the IMPs differently, suggesting that they are regulated independently of TIMP and from each other. The secretion of a battery of metalloproteinases by astrocytes may be important in facilitating astrocytic

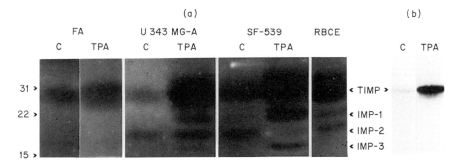

Figure 2. Secretion of metalloproteinase inhibitors by fetal astrocytes and cells from glioma cell lines. (a) Medium conditioned by fetal astrocytes (FA) or cells from glioma cell lines (U343 MG-A and SF-539), before (C) or after (TPA) treatment with 80 nM TPA, was analysed by reverse-gelatin zymography. Conditioned medium of TPA-treated RBCE was used as a standard to indicate the positions of TIMP, IMP-1, and IMP-2. The inhibitor positions (including IMP-3) are indicated at the right and molecular weight markers ($M_r \times 10^{-3}$) at the left. (b) U 343 MG-A cells were grown in serum-free Dulbecco's modified Eagle's medium in the absence (C) or presence (TPA) of 80 nM TPA for 48 h before being continuously labelled with [^{35}S]methionine. TIMP was immunoprecipitated with anti-TIMP IgG and analysed by autoradiography of SDS–polyacrylamide gels. The immunoprecipitated TIMP is marked at the left.

migration during development and in pathologic conditions such as inflammation or local invasion of astrocytic neoplasms. The regulation of metalloproteinase activity by the co-secretion of endogenous inhibitors may help explain certain features of the pathology of malignant gliomas, especially the rarity with which they metastasize.

Because the same metalloproteinases and their inhibitors are found associated with tumour cells and with cells involved in wound repair, it is likely that the mechanisms for connective tissue matrix turnover in tumours and wounds are similar. In this respect, tumours and wounds may differ only in the degree of regulation of proteolytic mechanisms.

CHARACTERIZATION OF IMP-2

IMP-2 (also known as TIMP-2) has been purified from medium conditioned by human fibroblasts (E.W. Howard and M.J. Banda, unpublished observations) and by human melanoma cells (Stetler-Stevenson *et al.*, 1989). A common feature of these purifications is the use of gelatin-affinity chromatography (Stetler-Stevenson *et al.*, 1989). When medium conditioned

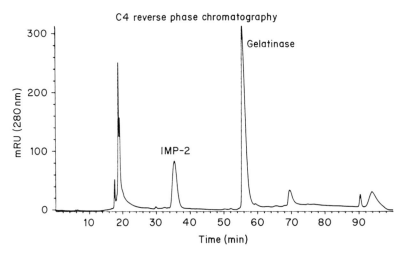

Figure 3. Separation of IMP-2 from gelatinases. Samples containing IMP-2 and gelatinase that eluted from a gelatin-affinity column were applied to a C4 reverse phase column equilibrated in 0.05% trifluoroacetic acid (TFA) at 0.5 ml/min. The column was developed with a linear gradient (0.3%/min) of 30% to 50% acetonitrile containing 0.05% TFA beginning at 15 min. Acetonitrile and TFA were removed from the collected fractions by rotary evaporation in a Speed-Vac. Fractions were reconstituted in aqueous buffer and analysed by reverse gelatin zymography.

by human fibroblasts (HS-395) was passed over a gelatin-affinity column, IMP-2 and the M_r 68 000 and M_r 92 000 gelatinases appeared to bind specifically to the column and elute together. IMP-2 was separated from the two proteinases by reverse phase chromatography (Fig. 3). When the resultant IMP-2, now free of proteinase, was reapplied to the gelatin-affinity column, it did not bind. This suggests that the original binding of IMP-2 to the column was the result of its being in complex with the pro-form of gelatinase that binds to gelatin. The pure IMP-2 is an effective inhibitor of the active form of the M_r 68 000 gelatinase (Stetler-Stevenson *et al.*, 1989). Because the gelatinase recovered from the dissociation of IMP-2: gelatinase complexes remains active, it is possible that IMP-2-mediated inhibition *in vivo* is reversible. Whether reversible inhibition is biologically relevant remains to be established. The degradation of type IV collagen and gelatin is inhibited at 1:1 molar ratio of IMP-2 and proteinase (Stetler-Stevenson *et al.*, 1989). Thus, IMP-2 can bind to both the pro- and active forms of M_r 68 000 gelatinase.

The amino terminal sequence of IMP-2 is similar to that of TIMP (Fig. 4) but does not match any sequence in TIMP. Therefore, IMP-2 is not a cleavage fragment of TIMP. The sequence similarity does, however, suggest that TIMP and IMP-2 may be part of a related family of proteinase inhibitors.

COMPARISON OF TIMP AND IMP-2

It is well established that both normal and tumour cells secrete a number of distinct but related metalloproteinases that are capable of degrading various components of the extracellular matrix. Recent data suggest that the same cells also secrete one or more distinct but related inhibitors of metallo-proteinases, the best characterized of which is TIMP. We have detected three other secreted inhibitors of metalloproteinases that we call IMPs. The amino terminal sequence of IMP-2 was determined during the present study. The entire amino acid sequence of IMP-2 (TIMP-2) was determined by Stetler-Stevenson *et al.* (1989). The amino terminal sequences are in

```
TIMP    C-T-C-V-P-P-H-P-Q-T-A-F-C-N-S-D-L-V-I-R-A-K-
IMP-2   C-S-C-S-P-V-H-P-Q-Q-A-F-C-N-A-D-V-V-I-R-A-K-
BCDI    C-S-C-S-P-V-H-P-Q-Q-A-F-C-N-A-C-I-V-I-R-A-K-
```

Figure 4. Comparison of the amino terminal sequences of human IMP-2 and human TIMP. After C4 reverse phase chromatography, IMP-2 was sequenced by automated gas phase Edman degradation. The sequence of TIMP was taken from Docherty *et al.*, 1985. The sequence of BCDI was taken from Murray *et al.* (1986).

agreement. Based on the entire amino acid sequence, TIMP and IMP-2 (TIMP-2) have 41% homology. This homology supports the contention that TIMP and IMP-2 are members of a related family of metalloproteinase inhibitors. The sequence of the bovine equivalent of IMP-2 has also been reported (Murray *et al.*, 1986; DeClerck *et al.*, 1989). This bovine molecule has been referred to as the bovine cartilage-derived inhibitor (BCDI; Murray *et al.*, 1986) and may be related to the cartilage-derived inhibitor of angiogenesis (Fig. 4). The identity of human IMP-2 with BCDI was confirmed with an antibody raised against BCDI that reacts with human IMP-2 but not with human TIMP (data not shown). Antibodies raised against human TIMP do not react with any of the three IMPs (Fig.2). These data suggest that the cartilage-derived inhibitor of angiogenesis and BCDI are IMP-2 and not TIMP.

The data gathered to date suggest that IMP-2 may preferentially inhibit at least the M_r 68 000 gelatinase. Until the kinetics of inhibition by IMP-2 and TIMP are determined for several metalloproteinases, the selectivity of these inhibitors cannot be determined. However, it should be noted that little if any TIMP bound to and eluted from the gelatin-affinity column described in this study. Therefore, TIMP may not be involved in the *in vivo* regulation of at least the M_r 68 000 gelatinase.

TIMP is an excellent inhibitor of interstitial collagenase (K_i less than 10^{-9}; Welgus *et al.*, 1985) with tight binding kinetics ($K_d = 1.4 \times 10^{-10}$; Cawston *et al.*, 1983). It is intriguing to speculate on the selectivity of TIMP versus IMP-2. Collagenase and stromelysin are structurally similar and may be preferentially inhibited by TIMP. In contrast, the two gelatinases are structurally similar and may be preferentially inhibited by IMP-2. It remains to be determined whether this speculation is supported by new data. However, it is proper to conclude that the degradation of extracellular matrix by metalloproteinases is regulated by more than simply the presence or absence of TIMP. As a family of metalloproteinases is involved in the turnover of matrix proteins during wound healing and angiogenesis, it is likely that a family of metalloproteinase inhibitors, of which TIMP and IMP-2 are members, is involved in the regulation of proteolysis.

ACKNOWLEDGEMENTS

We are grateful to Rick Lyman for help in preparing the manuscript and to Mary McKenney for editing it. We thank Karyn Bouhana and Elizabeth Bullen for technical assistance and acknowledge the collaborative efforts of James H. McKerrow on the astrocyte studies and Zena Werb on the RBCE studies. This work was supported by the Office of Health and Environmental

Research, US Department of Energy (contract no. DE-AC03-76-SF01012), a National Research Service Award from the NIEHS (5 T32 ES07106), and a grant from the National Institutes of Health (AR32746).

REFERENCES

Ausprunk, D.H. and Folkman, J. (1977). Migration and proliferation of endothelial cells in preformed and newly formed blood vessels during tumor angiogenesis. *Microvasc. Res.*, **14**, 53–65.

Bunning, R.A.D., Murphy, G., Kumar, S., Phillips, P. and Reynolds, J.J. (1984). Metalloproteinase inhibitors from bovine cartilage and body fluids. *Eur. J. Biochem.*, **139**, 75–80.

Burger, P.C., Chandler, D.B. and Klintworth, G.K. (1983). Corneal neovascularization as studied by scanning electron microscopy of vascular casts. *Lab. Invest.*, **48**, 169–180.

Cawston, T.E., Murphy, G., Mercer, E., Galloway, W.A., Hazleman, B.L. and Reynolds, J.J. (1983). The interaction of purified rabbit bone collagenase with purified rabbit bone metalloproteinase inhibitor. *Biochem. J.*, **211**, 313–318.

DeClerck, Y.A., Yean, T.-D., Ratzkin, B.J., Lu, H.S. and Langley, K.E. (1989). Purification and characterization of two related but distinct metalloproteinase inhibitors secreted by bovine aortic endothelial cells. *J. Biol. Chem.*, **264**, 17445–17453.

Docherty, A.J.P., Lyons, A., Smith, B.J., Wright, E.M., Stephens, P.E., Harris, T.J.R., Murphy, G. and Reynolds, J.J. (1985). Sequence of human tissue inhibitor of metalloproteinases and its identity to erythroid-potentiating activity. *Nature*, **318**, 66–69.

Folkman, J. (1984). What is the role of endothelial cells in angiogenesis? (Editorial). *Lab. Invest.*, **51**, 601–604.

Gavrilovic, J., Hembry, R.M., Reynolds, J.J. and Murphy, G. (1987). Tissue inhibitor of metalloproteinases (TIMP) regulates extracellular type I collagen degradation by chondrocytes and endothelial cells. *J. Cell. Sci.*, **87**, 357–362.

Herron, G.S., Banda, M.J., Clark, E.J., Gavrilovic, J. and Werb, Z. (1986a). Secretion of metalloproteinases by capillary endothelial cells. II. Expression of collagenase and stromelysin activities is regulated by endogenous inhibitors. *J. Biol. Chem.*, **261**, 2814–2818.

Herron, G.S., Werb, Z., Dwyer, K. and Banda, M.J. (1986b). Secretion of metalloproteinases by stimulated capillary endothelial cells. I. Production of procollagenase and prostromelysin exceeds expression of proteolytic activity. *J. Biol. Chem.*, **261**, 2810–2813.

Khokha, R., Waterhouse, P., Yagel, S., Lala, P.K., Overall, C.M., Norton, G. and Denhardt, D.T. (1989). Antisense RNA-induced reduction in murine TIMP levels confers oncogenicity on Swiss 3T3 cells. *Science*, **243**, 947–950.

Macartney, H.W. and Tschesche, H. (1983). The collagenase inhibitor from human polymorphonuclear leukocytes. Isolation, purification and characterisation. *Eur. J. Biochem.*, **130**, 79–83.

Mignatti, P., Robbins, E. and Rifkin, D.B. (1986). Tumor invasion through the human amniotic membrane: Requirements for a proteinase cascade. *Cell*, **47**, 487–498.

Murray, J.B., Allison, K., Sudhalter, J. and Langer, R. (1986). Purification and partial amino acid sequence of a bovine cartilage-derived collagenase inhibitor. *J. Biol. Chem.*, **261**, 4154–4159.

Stetler-Stevenson, W.G., Krutzsch, H.C. and Liotta, L.A. (1989). Tissue inhibitor of metalloproteinase (TIMP-2): A new member of the metalloproteinase inhibitor family. *J. Biol. Chem.*, **264**, 17374–17378.

Welgus, H.G., Jeffrey, J.J., Eisen, A.Z., Roswit, W.T. and Stricklin, G.P. (1985). Human skin fibroblast collagenase: interaction with substrate and inhibitor. *Coll. Relat. Res.*, **5**, 167–179.

Yasui, N., Hori, H. and Nagai, Y. (1981). Production of collagenase inhibitor by the growth cartilage of embryonic chick bone: isolation and partial characterization. *Coll. Relat. Res.*, **1**, 59–72.

Wound Healing
Edited by H. Janssen, R. Rooman and J.I.S. Robertson
© 1991 Wrightson Biomedical Publishing Ltd

8

Wound Healing: A Result of Coordinate Keratinocyte–Fibroblast Interactions. The Role of Keratinocyte Cytokines

J.F. NICOLAS, M. GAUCHERAND, E. DELAPORTE, D. HARTMAN[1], M. RICHARD[2], F. CROUTE and J. THIVOLET

Dermatology Clinic and Inserm U. 209, [2]Biochemistry Laboratory B, E. Herriot Hospital and [1]Radioanalysis Centre, Pasteur Institute, Lyon, France

Cellular interactions between epithelial (keratinocytes) and mesenchymal (fibroblasts) compartments appear to be of major importance for optimal differentiation of human skin during ontogeny (Briggaman, 1982; Woodley *et al.*, 1987). Similarly, intimate relationships between these two cell types are necessary for normal and complete wound repair (Alvarez *et al.*, 1987). Wound healing comprises a coordinated series of events occurring in the epidermis and the dermis leading to appropriate resurfacing (epitheliazation) together with replacement of the dermal defect (production of new connective tissue) (Clark, 1985). Fibroblasts are the main cell type responsible for the production of collagen and other extracellular matrix components. After tissue injury these cells are stimulated to proliferate and synthesize matrix constituents for repair. This fibroblast activation is controlled by numerous factors released by various cell types present in the lesion. The balance between stimulatory and inhibitory factors is responsible for the initiation and the termination of the wound healing process.

Although wound healing is a very complex series of phenomena involving many cell types and tissues (endothelial cells, blood mononuclear cells, epidermal and dermal cells) we want here to develop the concept that wound healing is primarily the result of the interaction between two cell types: keratinocytes and fibroblasts.

FIBROBLASTS PROMOTE KERATINOCYTE PROLIFERATION AND DIFFERENTIATION

Fibroblasts secrete various components of the extracellular matrix involved in epithelial cell (EC) growth and metabolism (Bohnert *et al.*, 1986; Woodley *et al.*, 1987). Fibronectin and laminin are indispensible for attachment and spreading of keratinocytes, whereas vinculin, fibronectin and glycosaminoglycans promote their migration. *In vitro*, the presence of fibroblasts used as feeder layers improves the proliferation and differentiation properties of EC, and this effect is probably related to soluble mediators (Green *et al.*, 1979). More importantly, when cultured epithelial sheets are grafted on to a partial thickness wound bed a complete differentiation of the grafted epithelium is obtained. Comparison of the cultured epidermis before and after grafting and analysis of keratins and various keratinocyte membrane antigens showed that full keratinocyte differentiation was only achieved after *in vivo* transplantation (Thivolet *et al.*, 1986). Thus, several observations argue for the role of fibroblasts and fibroblast products in the metabolism of epithelial cells.

KERATINOCYTES STIMULATE FIBROBLAST PROLIFERATION AND METABOLISM

Increasing evidence indicates that ECs are capable of releasing a variety of products endowed with immunoregulatory and metabolic activities (Kupper, 1989; Luger *et al.*, 1985; Sauder *et al.*, 1988) among which are interleukin-1/epidermal cell-derived thymocyte activation factor (IL-1/ETAF), IL-3, IL-6, granulocyte/macrophage-colony stimulating factor(GM-CSF), tumour necrosis factor-α (TNF-α) (Oxholm *et al.*, 1988), transforming growth factor-α (TGF-α) (Coffey *et al.*, 1987) and TGF-β (Gottlieb *et al.*, 1988) (Tables 1, 2 and 3). IL-1/ETAF is responsible for inducing fibroblast proliferation (Freundlich *et al.*, 1986; Schmidt *et al.*, 1982). It enhances type I and type III collagen mRNAs and proteins (Kahari *et al.*, 1987; Mauviel *et al.*, 1987) and increases collagenase production (Postlethwaite *et al.*, 1983). Recently human recombinant IL-1 has been shown to promote the healing of wounds in pigs (Mertz *et al.*, 1989). However, the role of keratinocytes in fibroblast metabolism remains poorly understood. One major criticism of the former studies, in respect to their physiological relevance, is that they are simple. These studies analyse the effect of just one defined product on a given variable. Moreover most of the studies involved synovial fibroblasts and chondrocytes and only a few concerned dermal human fibroblasts. Although such studies are of major importance they must be interpreted with caution especially when considering the *in vivo* relevance of this *in vitro* phenomenon. In this respect it is now well established that a given cell can produce

Table 1. Epidermal cytokines (interleukins).

	IL-1	Il-2	IL-3	IL-4	IL-5	IL-6	IL-7	IL-8
Source	Ubiq.[a]	Restr.[b]	Ubiq.	Restr.	Restr.	Ubiq.	?	?
Keratinocyte production	Yes	No	Yes	No	No	Yes	?	?

[a] Ubiquitous/several distinct cell types.
[b] Restricted mostly to T cells.

Table 2. Epidermal cytokines (colony stimulating factors, cytotoxins and growth factors).

Factors	Colony stimulating factors(CSF)				Cytotoxins (TNF-α)	Growth factors (TGF-α, β)
	Multi-CSF (IL-3)	GM-CSF	G-CSF	M-CSF		
Source	Ubiq.[a]	Ubiq.	Ubiq.	?	Ubiq.	Ubiq.
Keratinocyte production	Yes	Yes	?	?	Yes	Yes

[a] Ubiquitous/several cell types.

Table 3. Keratinocyte cytokines.

● IL-1 α, β (ETAF)
● Tumour necrosis factor-α
● IL-3 (multi-CSF)
● IL-6
● GM-CSF
● Transforming growth factor-α, β

simultaneously a given cytokine and a soluble factor able to inhibit the action of that cytokine. This is true for keratinocytes which constitutively release IL-1/ETAF and which can be driven to produce an IL-1 inhibitor under certain circumstances (Schwarz et al., 1987).

Our laboratory has been involved for several years in studying the role of keratinocytes in the normal development of dermal components, and especially in wound healing. Faure and coworkers have used autologous and allogenic cultured epidermal cells to recover different types of wounds, e.g. burns and venous ulcers. The results of these studies showed that grafting leads to a rapid healing of large wounds (Faure et al., 1987). Fibroblasts appeared to be stimulated to proliferate and synthesize extracellular matrix

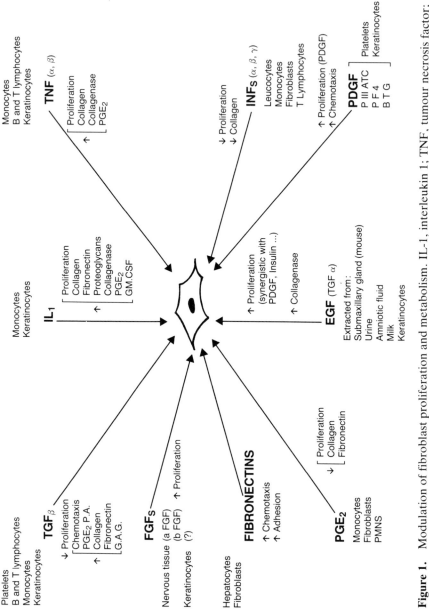

Figure 1. Modulation of fibroblast proliferation and metabolism. IL-1, interleukin 1; TNF, tumour necrosis factor; INF, interferons; PDGF, platelet-derived growth factor; EGF, epidermal growth factor; PGE₂, prostaglandin E₂; FGF, fibroblast growth factor; TGF, transforming growth factor.

components, leading to the reconstitution of a normal dermis. In such models (unlike other more classic procedures of skin grafting), the grafted tissue is exclusively composed of keratinocytes; therefore the resulting dermal repair of wounds observed must be attributed to epithelial cells and epithelial cell products.

HETEROGENEITY OF THE KERATINOCYTE-DERIVED FACTORS INVOLVED IN FIBROBLAST PROLIFERATION

Based on the *in vivo* observation discussed above we decided to study more precisely the *in vitro* effect of keratinocytes on fibroblasts. We focused on the effect of soluble factors produced by keratinocytes on two major functions of fibroblasts during wound healing: proliferation and production of collagen. Considering that fibroblasts are exposed *in vivo* to a large array of keratinocyte products we preferred testing crude keratinocyte culture supernatants rather than individual and well characterized cytokines.

The experimental protocol was as follows: conditioned media from 48 hour cultures of subconfluent normal keratinocytes (normal human keratinocytes, human and murine keratinocyte cell lines) were added to normal human dermal fibroblasts. Fibroblast proliferation was measured using a Coulter counter and collagen type I and type III was quantified by radioimmunoassay using antibodies specific for human collagen type I and type III.

The first major observation was that keratinocytes were potent stimulators of fibroblast growth through the production of soluble factors (Delaporte *et al.*, 1989a). Biochemical analysis of epidermal cell culture supernatants (by gel filtration chromatography) revealed three fractions corresponding to M_r of 10, 18, and 21 K endowed with the stimulatory activity. Considering the molecular mass range of these factors the question of their relationship to known keratinocyte-derived cytokines, and especially to IL-1, was raised. IL-1 is a 17.5 kDa pleiotropic cytokine, constitutively produced by keratinocytes (Oppenheim *et al.*, 1986). That IL-1 induces fibroblast proliferation was demonstrated using the purified as well as the recombinant human molecule and this property has been used in the past for IL-1 titration in biological fluids. Our keratinocyte culture supernatants and gel filtration fractions contained detectable quantities of IL-1, suggesting that the stimulatory factor could be IL-1 itself.

However, several observations argue against the hypothesis of IL-1 being the only molecule responsible for fibroblast proliferation. First, recombinant human IL-1 was 1.5–2 times less efficient than keratinocyte culture supernatants in stimulation of fibroblast growth. Second, no correlation was found between IL-1 production by different keratinocyte cell types and their ability to stimulate fibroblast growth; in this respect, PAM cells which exhibited the highest stimulatory index produced less IL-1 than the two other keratinocyte cell types. Third, absorption of IL-1 activity in our samples was not associated with abolition of the stimulatory activity; preincubation of conditioned media or column fractions with antibodies to IL-1-α and β resulted in only a 50% inhibition in fibroblast growth. These results suggested that keratinocytes produce several types of soluble factors involved in fibroblast proliferation, one of these factors being IL-1. In our hands, human rIL-3 and rGM-CSF did not modify proliferation of dermal fibroblasts. Furthermore, no IL-6 or GM-CSF could be detected in active fractions endowed with high stimulatory activity. Thus, none of these three epidermal cytokines seems to be involved in the activity described here.

Epidermal cells synthesize a number of soluble factors that could stimulate (IL-1 (Schmidt *et al.*, 1982), TNF-α (Vilcek *et al.*, 1986), PDGF) or inhibit (anti-IL-1, PGE2) fibroblast growth (Table 4). Little is known about the amount of each factor produced by EC *in vivo* or *in vitro* and most of the studies now utilize mRNA expression as a parameter. However mRNA expression does not necessarily correlate with protein synthesis and release since post-transcriptional regulatory events can occur. This applies to the recent demonstration of mRNAs for TGF-α and β and TNF-α in human and mouse keratinocytes (Gottlieb *et al.*, 1988). Whether TNF and TGF molecules are released by EC in biologically active quantities and have implications in fibroblast growth remains to be shown.

Table 4.   Cytokines affecting fibroblast growth.

Stimulation
- IL-1
- Tumour necrosis factor (TNF)
- Platelet-derived growth factor (PDGF)
- Epidermal growth factor (EGF)
- Fibroblast growth factor (FGF)

Inhibition
- Interferons (α, γ)
- Transforming growth factor (TGF) β
- PGE$_2$

EFFECT OF KERATINOCYTE-DERIVED SOLUBLE FACTORS ON COLLAGEN PRODUCTION BY NORMAL DERMAL HUMAN FIBROBLASTS

Using a similar experimental protocol we tested the effect of keratinocyte-derived molecules on collagen type I and type III production by human fibroblasts. We demonstrated that keratinocyte-derived soluble factors stimulate total (I+III) collagen production by 10–40%. In addition, collagen production was unaffected by IL-1-β, IL-2, IL-3 and GM-CSF (Delaporte *et al.*, 1989b). That Il-1, which is a potent stimulator of collagen mRNA production (Kahari *et al.*, 1987), did not in our hands induce an increase in soluble collagen production appeared more surprising. However, Duncan and Berman (1989) recently reported that differential effects of IL-1 on collagen production could be obtained depending on the absence or the presence of FCS in the culture medium. IL-1 induced stimulation of collagen production, and secretion was achieved only in the absence of FCS; addition of FCS resulted in an apparent lack of stimulation of collagen synthesis. Our experiments were all performed with 5% FCS and thus our results are in agreement with those of Duncan and Berman.

The second part of the results concerned the differential expression of type I and type III collagen by two different fibroblast cell lines (F1 and F2) upon stimulation by keratinocyte-derived soluble factors. The F1 cell line responded to stimulation with keratinocyte soluble factors with a 350% increase in collagen type III secretion, whereas no modification in collagen type I production was seen. Alternatively the response of F2 fibroblasts to the same keratinocyte conditioned media consisted in a moderate increase (20–30%) of both collagen type I and type III. From these results we conclude that type I and type III collagen production is controlled by distinct regulatory mechanisms or molecular entities present in keratinocyte culture supernates. This result appears somewhat surprising considering that modulators of collagen production have been reported to affect both type I and type III collagen (Postlethwaite *et al.*, 1984). The reasons for this discrepancy are presently not known. None of the recombinant human cytokines used were able to modify significantly type I or type III collagen production by any of the two fibroblast cell lines.

REGULATION OF WOUND HEALING

As developed above, keratinocyte products could by themselves induce fibroblast activation, proliferation and synthesis of extracellular matrix proteins (Tables 4 and 5). Furthermore, keratinocyte cytokines are able to stimulate collagenase production by fibroblasts (via Il-1 and TNF) (Dayer *et al.*, 1985; Duncan and Berman, 1989) and this phenomenon is probably involved in the regulation of dermal repair. It is obvious that after a phase of stimulation of fibroblast metabolism (anabolic phase) there must be a phase where fibroblast activation is switched off and even a catabolic phase leading to a remodelling of the extracellular matrix by collagenases, glycosaminogly-canases and elastases.

Table 5.   Cytokines affecting collagen synthesis.

Stimulation
- IL-1 (w/o FCS)
- TGF
- TNF
- Collagen stimulating protein (100–170 kDa)

Inhibition
- PGE_2
- Interferons

Our experimental system comprising subconfluent pure keratinocyte cultures could be a good model of the first stages of wound healing. We have shown that the effect of keratinocyte-derived factors on fibroblasts was of the anabolic type. It is possible that during wound healing, when epithelial cells recover the wound totally and start to differentiate, modifications occur in the production of cytokines which then could inhibit fibroblast proliferation and collagen production.

Interferons (IFN), especially γ-IFN, are one of the potential candidates of the down-regulation of cytokine-induced fibroblast activation. γ-Interferon, a product of activated CD^{4+} cells, inhibits collagen production (Melin et al., 1989; Postlethwaite et al., 1983), and these CD^{4+} cells are found in situ in wounds at an early stage (Morhenn, 1988). The hypothesis that products of inflammatory cells modulate fibroblast metabolism and wound healing has been discussed for a long time and was reviewed recently (Morhenn, 1988; Perlish and Fleischmayer, 1989), Wound fluid, which contains plasma and soluble factors secreted by the infiltrating cells is a potent inhibitor of fibroblast growth (Bucalo et al., 1989). Thus, it is apparent that the various cells of the skin and their soluble products interact in a complex way. Recent developments of in vitro models able to test these interactions better (Krueger et al., 1989) will bring new insights to the comprehension of wound healing.

REFERENCES

Alvarez, O.M., Golsen, J.B., Eaglstein, W.H., Welgus, H.G. and Stricklin, G.P. (1987). Wound Healing. In: Fitzpatrick, T.B. (Ed.), *Dermatology in General Medicine*, McGraw Hill, New York, pp. 321–336.
Bohnert, A., Hornung, J. and Mackenzie, I.C. (1986). Epithelial–mesenchymal interactions control basement membrane production and differentiation in cultured and transplanted mouse keratinocytes. *Cell Tissue Res.*, **244**, 413–429.

Briggaman, R.A. Epidermal–dermal interactions in adult skin. *J. Invest. Dermatol.*, **79**, 21S–24S.

Bucalo, B., Eaglstein, W.H. and Falanga, V. (1989). The effect of chronic wound fluid on cell proliferation. *J. Invest. Dermatol.*, **92**, 408A.

Clark, R.A.F. (1985). Cutaneous tissue repair: I–basic biologic considerations, II–practical implications of current knowledge. *J. Am. Acad. Dermatol.*, **13**, 701–725; 919–941.

Coffey, R.J., Derinck, R., Wilcox, J.R., Bringman, T.S., Goustin, A.S., Moses, H.L. and Pittelkow, M.R. (1987). Production and auto-induction of transforming growth factor alpha in human keratinocytes. *Nature*, **328**, 817–820.

Dayer, J.M., Beutler, B. and Cerami, A. (1985). Cachectin/tumor necrosis factor stimulates collagenase and prostaglandin E2 production by human synovial cells and dermal fibroblasts. *J. Exp. Med.*, **162**, 632–643.

Delaporte, E., Nicolas, J.F., Bonnefoy, J.Y., Croute, F., Robert, J. and Thivolet, J. (1989a). Normal human keratinocytes produce soluble factors stimulating fibroblast proliferation *in vitro*. Relationship to keratinocyte cytokines. *J. Invest. Dermatol.*, **92**, 419A.

Delaporte, E., Hartman, D.J., Croute, F., Robert, J., Thivolet, J. and Nicolas, J.F. (1989b). Keratinocyte–fibroblast interactions. II. Stimulation of fibroblast type I and type III collagen production by epidermal cytokines. *J. Invest. Dermatol.*, **92**, 138A.

Duncan, M.R. and Berman, B. (1989). Differential regulation of collagen, glycosaminoglycan, fibronectin and collagenase activity production in cultured human adult fibroblasts by interleukin-1 alpha and beta and tumor necrosis factor alpha and beta. *J. Invest. Dermatol.*, **92**, 699–706.

Faure, M., Mauduit, G., Schmitt, D., Kanitakis, J., Demidem, A. and Thivolet, J. (1987). Growth and differentiation of human epidermal cultures used as auto and allografts in humans. *Brit. J. Dermatol.*, **116**, 161–170.

Fleitschmayer, R., Perlish, J.S. and Duncan, M. (1983). Scleroderma. A model for fibrosis. *Arch. Dermatol.*, **119**, 957–962.

Freundlich, B., Bomalaski, J.S., Neilson, E. and Jimenez, S.A. (1986). Regulation of fibroblast proliferation and collagen synthesis by cytokines. *Immunol. Today*, **7**, 303–307.

Gottlieb, A.B., Khong Chang, C., Posnett, D.N., Fanelli, B. and Tam, J.M. (1988). Detection of transforming growth factor alpha in normal, malignant, and hyperproliferative human keratinocytes. *J. Exp. Med.*, **167**, 670–675.

Green, H., Kehinde, O. and Thomas, J. (1989). Growth of cultural human epidermal cells into multiple epithelia suitable for grafting. *Proc. Natl Acad. Sci. (USA)*, **76**, 5665–5668.

Kahari, V.M., Heino, J. and Vuorio, E. (1987). Interleukin-1 increases collagen production and mRNA levels in cultured skin fibroblasts. *Biochem. Biophys. Acta.*, **929**, 142–147.

Krueger, G.G., Jorgensen, C.M., Bradshaw, B.R., Wall, L.L., Park, S.D. and Roberts, L.K. (1989). Approach for and assessment of interactive communication via cytokines of cellular constituents of the skin. *Dermatologica*, **179**, (Suppl. 1) 91–100.

Kupper, T.S. (1989). Production of cytokines by epithelial tissues. A new model for cutaneous inflammation. *Am. J. Dermatopathol.*, **11**, 69–73.

Luger, T.A., Kock, A., Danner, M., Colot, M. and Micksche, M. (1985). Production of distinct cytokines by epidermal cells. *Brit. J. Dermatol.*, **113**, (Suppl. 28), 145–156.

Mauviel, A., Bhatnagar, R., Penformis, H., Loyau, G., Saklatvala, J. and Pujol, J.P. (1987). Collagen production in synoviocytes cultured with interleukin-1. *J. Leuk. Biol.*, **42**, 557A.

Melin, M., Hartman, D.J., Magloire, H., Falcoff, E., Auriault, C. and Grimaud, J.A. (1989). Human recombinant gamma-interferon stimulates proliferation and inhibits collagen and fibronectin production by human dental pulp fibroblasts. *Cell. Mol. Biol.*, **35**, 97–110.

Mertz, P.M., Davis, S.C., Eaglstein, W.H., Kilian, P. and Sauder, D.N. (1989). Interleukin-1 is a potent inducer of wound reepithelialization. *J. Invest. Dermatol.*, **92**, 480A.

Morhenn, V. (1988). Keratinocyte proliferation in wound healing and skin diseases. *Immunol. Today*, **9**, 104–107.

Oppenheim, J.J., Kovacs, E.J., Matsushima, K. and Durum, S.K. (1986). There is more than one interleukin 1. *Immunol. Today*, **7**, 45–56.

Oxholm, A., Oxholm, P., Staberg, B. and Bendtzen, K. (1988). Immunohistological detection of interleukin 1-like molecules and tumor necrosis factor in human epidermis before and after UVB-irradiation *in vivo*. *Br. J. Dermatol.*, **118**, 369–376.

Perlish, J.S. and Fleischmayer, R. (1989). Immunologic stimulation of dermal fibroblasts in scleroderma. In: Norris, D.A. (Ed.), *Immune mechanisms in Cutaneous Diseases*, Marcel Dekker, New York, pp. 605–624.

Postlethwaite, A.E., Lachman, L.B., Mainardi, C.L. and Kang, A.H. (1983). Interleukin-1 stimulation of collagenase production by cultured fibroblasts. *J. Exp. Med.*, **157**, 801–806.

Postlethwaite, A.E., Smith, G.N., Mainardi, C.N., Seyer, J.M. and Kang, A.H. (1984). Lymphocyte modulation of fibroblast function *in vitro*: stimulation and inhibition of collagen production by different effector molecules. *J. Immunol.*, **132**, 2470–2477.

Sauder, D.N. (1988). Biologic properties of epidermal cell thymocyte activating factor (ETAF). *J. Invest. Dermatol.*, **85**, 176S–182S.

Schmidt, J.A., Mizel, S.B., Cohen, D. and Green, I. (1982). Interleukin 1: a potential regulator of fibroblast proliferation. *J. Immunol.*, **128**, 2177–2182.

Schwarz, T., Urbanski, A., Gschnait, F. and Luger, T.A. (1987). UV-irradiated epidermal cells produce a specific inhibitor of interleukin 1 activity. *J. Immunol.*, **138**, 1457–1463.

Thivolet, J., Faure, M., Demidem, A. and Maudit, G. (1986). Long term survival and immunological tolerance of human epidermal allografts produced in culture. *Transplantation*, **42**, 274–280.

Vilcek, J., Palombella, V.J., Hendriksen-Destefano, D., Swenson, C., Feinman, R., Hirai, M. and Tsujimoto, M. (1986). Fibroblast growth enhancing activity of tumor necrosis factor and its relationship to other polypeptide growth factors. *J. Exp. Med.*, **163**, 632–643.

Woodley, D.T., Demarchez, M., Sengel, P. and Prunieras, M. (1987). The control of cutaneous development and behaviour: the influence of extracellular and soluble factors. In: Fitzpatrick, T.B. (Ed.), *Dermatology in General Medicine*, McGraw Hill, New York, pp. 132–146.

Wound Healing
Edited by H. Janssen, R. Rooman and J.I.S. Robertson
© 1991 Wrightson Biomedical Publishing Ltd

9

The Response of Experimental Wounds to Endogenous and Exogenous Growth Factors

JEFFREY M. DAVIDSON and KENNETH N. BROADLEY

Department of Pathology, Vanderbilt University School of Medicine and Veterans Administration Medical Center, Nashville, Tennessee, USA

Over the past decade a body of experimental evidence has accumulated to suggest that growth promoting substances, known as cytokines or cellular growth factors, can successfully accelerate the course of wound repair (Davidson and Woodward, 1989; Clark and Henson, 1988; Barbul *et al.*, 1988). In a limited number of cases, these observations have gone on to the development of clinical trials (Brown *et al.*, 1989). The results of these trials may in fact result in the practical application of wound repair studies within a short time. This discussion will principally focus on the contributions that our own laboratory has made to developing, analysing and quantifying the effects of a variety of growth factors on the wound repair process in experimental animals. It is only reasonable to point out that this work does not establish any single growth factor or even combinations of growth factors as being optimal for the repair process. Indeed these studies emphasize the redundancy of wound repair mechanisms and the spectrum of mediators which can become involved at various stages of the process.

STAGES IN WOUND REPAIR

For discussion purposes it is useful to visualize wound repair as a series of overlapping organizational phases, beginning with clot formation and clot retraction (in the case of traumatic wounds), proceeding through the development of granulation tissue (a histological entity consisting of abundant blood vessels, loosely-organized fibroblastic cells and a mono-nuclear component), and finally proceeding to the stage of healing or scar formation in which collagen and other fibrillar connective tissue components come to dominate the wound site. Repair of different types of wounds can be different. Our studies have taken the premise that the rate of granulation tissue formation may be the critical step in repair of many of these wounds, since it is granulation tissue which assures a rich blood supply to the wound site and which is responsible for the deposition of extracellular matrix. There are semantic and operational differences between the terms 'granulating wounds' and 'granulation tissue', but at the microscopic level, these are indistinguishable.

THE SPONGE MODEL

The principal quantitative model we have employed in these studies has involved the implantation of a small polyvinyl alcohol (PVA) sponge of precise dimensions and weight beneath the ventral panniculus carnosus of the rat at four to six separate sites (Woodward and Herrman, 1968). Granulation tissue forms rapidly within the interstices of this sponge, replacing the initial fibrin clot that arises from a plasma exudate. Organization of granulation tissue proceeds in an inwardly radial fashion allowing one to evaluate subjectively the degree of organization and penetration in histological specimens. A wide variety of other so-called 'dead space' models are available (Davidson and Woodward, 1989). We find the PVA sponge system to be highly reproducible, with complete filling of the sponge taking about 14 days in a normal rat at which time collagen content and DNA content reach a maximum value. The sponges are well suited for biochemical analysis: DNA content, protein content, and collagen content, measured as hydroxyproline. RNA isolation is also straightforward using SDS-proteinase K extraction (Sambrook et al., 1989). Using this kind of experimental system, one can demonstrate that many substances, both defined and undefined, that are introduced into the interstices of the sponge matrix will accelerate the rate of granulation tissue formation. The challenge to investigators is defining the mechanisms by which this stimulation occurs.

Our initial exploitation of this system showed for the first time that epidermal growth factor (EGF) would produce an acceleration of granulation tissue formation only if presented as a continuously released substance (Buckley et al., 1985; 1987). In concurrent studies, we applied the model to another cytokine, basic fibroblast growth factor (bFGF) which proved to cause an acceleration of granulation tissue formation but after only a single dose (Davidson et al., 1985), suggesting that these two cytokines operated through very different cellular recognition and response mechanisms.

INCISIONAL MODEL

The second model which we have used over the past several years, is the traditional incisional healing model in the rat. This model may be a more widely accepted measure of wound healing, at least by surgeons. Incisional models are far less accessible to biochemical analysis but provide quantitative data on tensile properties of wounds and histologic information on the quality of reorganization of connective tissue at the incision site. Using such a model, we have recently shown that bFGF has a mild, positive effect on incisional strength only early in the repair process (McGee *et al.*, 1988), whereas transforming growth factor-β (TGF-β) (McGee *et al.*, 1989; also a single dose) produced large, persistent, increasing strengthening of experimental incisional wounds. Similar but less persistent effects were reported by Mustoe *et al.* (1987).

GROWTH FACTORS

At present, there is a whirlwind of activity in the cytokine field. Historically EGF and its receptor had served as prototypes for growth factor action, but it is now clear that growth factors can differ widely in their specific effects on cells and tissues. The growth factors with which we have had the greatest amount of experience can be grouped into three families. EGF has a close structural relationship to TGF-α (Derynck, 1986). The latter may be more widely expressed during development and disease than EGF *per se*. They are both low molecular weight polypeptides (M_r 6000) that interact with a single 170 kDa cell surface receptor having tyrosine kinase activity. Indeed, all of the cellular growth factors seem to share the property of kinase activity; therefore it is still quite unclear how the specificity of signalling, that is recognition of kinase substrate, is generated within the cell.

The second class of growth factors has as its prototype type bFGF. This factor together with acidic fibroblast growth factor were originally isolated from pituitary extracts, but these factors (particularly bFGF) are widely distributed in tissues (Rifkin and Moscatelli, 1989). FGFs often associate with the extracellular matrix as the result of their strong affinity for heparin sulphate. This growth factor family now consists of at least seven members, all sharing high affinity for heparin. Although bFGF can be synthesized in several molecular forms (Rifkin and Moscatelli, 1989). there is a paradoxical lack of a signal peptide in bFGF, raising questions about the manner in which this hormone reaches other cells. *In vitro*, however, wounded endothelial cells will release a bFGF-like molecule (McNeil *et al.*, 1989; Sato and Rifkin, 1988) and cells transfected with bFGF cDNA coupled to a signal peptide will produce an extracellular matrix that possesses FGF-like activity (Rogelj *et al.*,

1988). EGF and TGF-α have a broad capacity to stimulate cell growth both in mesenchymal and epithelial cells. In contrast, bFGF is an especially strong mitogen for endothelial cells, which probably contributes to its angiogenic activity.

A third class of growth factors is represented by TGF-β1, one of at least five homologous gene products present in mammals and further related to other molecules such as activin and Mullerian inhibitory substance (Sporn *et al.*, 1987). The name TGF-β is a misnomer, since this potent cytokine is a significant growth inhibitor for most normal cells. The remarkable property of this molecule is stimulation of extracellular matrix production. High affinity receptors for TGF-β fall into three different size classes (Massague, 1987). TGF-β can be an extremely potent stimulus; for example it is reported to have chemotactic activity for mononuclear cells at femtomolar concentrations.

Each of these growth factors, EGF/TGF-α, bFGF, and TGF-β, has been shown to accelerate wound healing under appropriate experimental conditions (Davidson and Woodward, 1989). To summarize our own experimental findings we can say that EGF/TGF-α appears to act largely through mitogenic and chemotactic activity. There is sparse evidence to suggest that either can directly stimulate growth of new blood vessels or alter the rate of accumulation of connective tissue. EGF/TGF-α appears to promote repair by increasing the number of connective tissue cells within a wound site. bFGF, on the other hand, has different properties. It is a potent mitogen and chemoattractant for both mesenchymal and endothelial cells (Buckley-Sturrock *et al.*, 1989). The granulation tissue produced by bFGF is far richer in vascular elements, including widely dilated capillaries. In recent studies, in which bFGF has been continuously released into PVA sponges, one can produce an overwhelming angiogenic response, without reducing the production of other associated connective tissue elements, as is normally seen with a single injection of bFGF directly into the sponge. bFGF can also affect wound repair processes through its capacity to induce or modulate the expression of tissue proteinases, including plasminogen activator, collagenase and stromelysin. Thus, it is characteristic of bFGF-treated granulation tissue that increased cellularity is achieved at the expense of collagen content. TGF-β stimulates granulation tissue in a variety of ways. It is a potent chemoattractant and is likely to be involved in the recruitment of monocytes to the wound site, thereby stimulating the release of mononuclear or macrophage-derived cytokines. Secondly, it can produce markedly increased expression of extracellular matrix molecules (two to five-fold) including the interstitial collagens, fibronectin, elastin and proteoglycans. Tissue proteinase expression is reduced. The predominant effect of TGF-β in the granulation tissue model is the accumulation of connective tissue, with little increase in cellularity or even a small reduction. These facts are quite consistent with its *in vitro* effect on cultured fibroblasts. Due to the remarkable stimulation of matrix formation, TGF-β has very strong effect on strengthening of incisional wounds (Mustoe *et al.*, 1987; McGee *et al.*, 1989; Pierce *et al.*, 1989). Granulation tissue is also more abundant in TGF-β treated incisions.

Recently with the help of Genentech we have evaluated TGF-β in an excisional wound model in the pig. This model does include an epidermal component. Our findings are consistent with results in the sponge model, namely that granulation tissue formation is accelerated in these wounds. We observed a mild transient retardation of epidermal overgrowth at high doses of TGF-β (Quaglino *et al.*, 1989a).

ENDOGENOUS CYTOKINES

Premises of all growth factor wound healing studies are first that these molecules are intrinsically involved in the repair process and second that one or several of the growth factors may be critical to the healing of wounds. This is based on several observations. First of all, platelet degranulation results in the release of a large bolus of growth factors including platelet derived growth factor (PDGF) and TGF-β. Concentrations of these molecules rise rapidly at wound sites after injury. Subsequently, others report expression of other PDGF-like molecules by the cells present at the wound site as well as increasing expression and accumulation of TGF-β. (Grotendorst *et al.*, 1988). It is postulated that the macrophage is the principal source of growth factors during the repair process, as evidenced by studies showing its capacity to express a range of growth factor genes and growth factor proteins (Rapolee *et al.*, 1988). Studies by ourselves and others have shown by immunolocalization or by *in situ* hybridization that a very restricted subset of mononuclear cells within the wound are expressing growth factors (Quaglino *et al.*, 1989a). Further support for this concept comes from findings that animals treated with either steroids or other immunosuppresive agents such as adriamycin manifest reduced numbers of monocytes and other bone-marrow-derived cells which normally deliver growth factors in the wound site.

Recently we have attempted to implicate more directly the growth factors in the repair process. Using monospecific polyclonal antisera directed against bFGF, we were able to show that the rate of organization and the accompanying biochemical parameters of wound healing were significantly retarded by the continuous release of these neutralizing antibodies into sponge granulation tissue (Broadley *et al.*, 1989a). These studies appear to be the first direct evidence that growth factors are rate-limiting to wound repair, and it is hoped that similar studies can be developed for other polypeptide cytokines as well.

IMPAIRED HEALING

An important realization in wound repair research is that normal, experimental animals heal at near-optimal rates and significant stimulation of wound repair by growth factors is difficult to obtain. Since one object of the study of growth factors is their potential application as promoters of wound healing, whether they will be cutaneous, vascular or orthopaedic, we have used several models to create or mimic situations in which wound healing proceeds at reduced rates. One convenient and cost-effective model is the streptozotocin-induced model of diabetes in the rat. While not an accurate model of the chronic human disease, since the diabetes is left uncontrolled and hyperglycaemia is extreme, the non-fatal condition promotes or sustains the presence of non-healing wounds. Both the rate of granulation tissue formation and the development of incisional strength are severely retarded, as shown by earlier work of others. The usefulness of this model has been the greater relative response of tissue to growth factors in the diabetic system. This holds for both granulation tissue and incisional wound in the case of TGF-β and for granulation tissue with respect to bFGF (Broadley et al., 1989b). Even greater improvement was obtained in diabetic rats by using a combination of these two factors. We find that combinations of bFGF and TGF-β can restore the parameters of wound repair to virtually normal levels, confirming the concept that cocktails of growth factor combinations should be considered seriously.

Other models which may be more physiologically relevant have been tested in our laboratory. The pig excisional wound is an accepted model of the full or partial-thickness injury. We have used glucocorticoid treatment to retard repair, as have other investigators using rats and other experimental animals. Positive effects of growth factors are more clearly delineated in the retarded-healing model. Chronological ageing is also felt to have an important impact on the repair process. We have extensively (and expensively) evaluated wound repair processes and the impact of growth factors in an ageing rat model sponsored by the National Institute on Aging (Quaglino et al., 1989b). Several important observations are developing. Studying a series of ages it was obvious that the 200 g (2 months old) rat is a very poor subject for wound repair studies, having an extremely high rate of wound repair. We strongly encourage investigators to use animals which are not juvenile, 400 g (4 months old) in the case of the Sprague–Dawley or Fisher 344 rats. We found that through most of adult life there was little change in the rate of wound repair with either sponge or incisional systems. However, in the last 20% of the rat lifespan (>25 months) granulation tissue organization and incisional strength were significantly reduced. In contrast to the findings in other impairment models, it has been difficult to obtain a marked growth factor response suggesting that there are several defective response mechanisms in aged animals.

CELLULAR MECHANISM

In order to understand which growth factors may be appropriate in a given wound healing environment, we require more detailed evidence of their *in vivo* action. A large fraction of our research effort has gone into attempts to describe the mechanism of action of growth factors. Perhaps the most graphic demonstration has come from a series of studies performed with D. Quaglino and L.B. Nanney, in which both rat granulation tissue and pig incisional wounds have been evaluated for local effects on gene expression by the method of *in situ* hybridization. Topical or injected TGF-β was used as a stimulus. Our findings show that, consistent with cell culture studies and recent reports of Pierce *et al.* (1989), collagen type I, collagen type III, elastin, and fibronectin expression are markedly accelerated by TGF-β treatment whereas stromelysin, a metalloproteinase thought to be representative of tissue metalloproteinase involved in matrix turnover, was sharply reduced (Quaglino *et al.*, 1989a). This observation would be consistent with the observed increases in matrix accumulation coming from a combination of increased synthesis of various matrix proteins and reduced degradation. A more novel and possibly more important finding in these studies was the observation that TGF-β increased expression of its own gene product, both in the degree of expression per cell and the number of cells within the wound expressing TGF-β. This may explain how single doses of the growth factor produce such profound and persistent effects.

At the cellular level, growth factors have a wide variety of effects on cells from the wound. Both EGF and bFGF have strong chemotactic properties for wound fibroblasts, thus accounting for increased cellularity as much through cell migration as increases in cell proliferation (Buckley-Sturrock *et al.*, 1989). In addition, our studies have shown that bFGF is a potent inducer of collagenase expression in wound tissue cells. Cytokine responses provide evidence of a changing phenotype among that fibroblast population since induction of collagenase was absent in populations of granulation tissue fibroblasts from mature wounds.

We have also been attempting to describe the phenotype of the wound fibroblast in terms of other cytokine responses. Following the observations of Bell *et al.* (1979) and Montesano and Orci (1988) T. Finesmith in our laboratory has performed experiments in which either TGF-β alone, bFGF alone, or the two cytokines in combination were used to challenge both normal rat skin fibroblasts and fibroblasts isolated from rat granulation tissue explanted at various stages of wound maturity (Finesmith *et al.*, 1989). In addition to confirming the observations of Montesano and Orci on what is felt to be a myofibroblast cell population, these studies have shown that both endogenous contractility and responsiveness to TGF-β increase in cells as the wound matures. In contrast, bFGF antagonizes the basal contractility of fibroblasts in a collagen gel. Furthermore, pretreatment of cells with bFGF, followed by exposure of cells to both TGF-β and bFGF, markedly reduced the stimulated contraction of the gel. These findings are consistent with the concept that bFGF alters the responses of cells to TGF-β, perhaps by down-regulation of TGF-β receptor. From this and several other studies in our laboratory comes the suggestion that the use of combinations of growth factors can adjust the response of cells and tissues to produce more optimal wound healing responses. For example, the combination of angiogenesis and fibrogenesis is essential to wound healing; agents which accelerate each of these processes can produce a synergistic effect. A further development of this approach would be to consider sequential application of different cytokines to the wound, mimicking the natural process.

CONCLUSIONS

Wound healing is an extremely complicated biological process. In some ways wound repair is a frustrated attempt by the organism to recapitulate selected developmental events: first, to re-establish tissue integrity and, secondly, to re-establish tissue function. The study of cutaneous or subcutaneous wounds may be the simplest experimental way to approach this problem since the evaluation of cell populations grown over many generations in tissue culture may have very little relationship to the complexity of interactions occurring in a three-dimensional matrix within the organism. One can use model wound systems in a variety of ways. First of all, models are useful for demonstrating preclinical efficacy of vulnerary substances. Such studies are scarcely limited to cytokines, as there are many other kinds of mediators that can promote the process. Secondly, experimental wound systems probably represent a tissue injury model that can be used to establish the relative and sequential influence of cytokines on the quality and quantity of repair. Thirdly, wound repair is an exciting and relevant paradigm for developing and refining our concepts of cell differentiation, the definition of phenotype and the regulation of gene expression. As the wound healing discipline matures over the next decade we feel confident that it can make major contributions, not only in the clinical arena, but in more basic issues of cellular and molecular biology.

ACKNOWLEDGEMENTS

Supported in part by grants from the National Institute on Aging (AG06528), Synergen, Inc., and Genentech, Inc.

REFERENCES

Barbul, A., Pines, E., Caldwell, M. and Hunt, T.K. (Eds) (1988). *Growth Factors and Other Aspects of Wound Healing*, Alan R. Liss, New York.

Bell, E., Ivarsson, B. and Merrill, C. (1979). Production of a tissue-like structure by contraction of collagen lattices by human fibroblasts of different proliferation potential *in vivo*. *Proc. Natl Acad. Sci. (USA).*, **76**, 1274–1278.

Broadley, K.N., Aquino, A.M., Woodward, S.C., Sturrock, A., Sato, Y., Rifkin, D.B. and Davidson, J.M. (1989a). Monospecific antibodies indicate that basic fibroblast growth factor is intrinsically involved in wound repair. *Lab. Invest.*, **61**, 571–575.

Broadley, K.N., Aquino, A.M., Hicks, B., Ditesheim, J.A., McGee, G.S., Demetriou, A.A., Woodward, S.C. and Davidson, J.M. (1989b). The diabetic rat is an impaired wound healing model: stimulatory effects of transforming growth factor-β and basic fibroblast growth factor. *Biotech. Therap.*, **1**, 55–68.

Brown, G.L., Nanney, L.B., Griffen, J., Cramer, A.B., Yancey, J.M., Curtsinger, L.J., Holtzin, L., Schultz, G.S., Jurkiewicz, M.J. and Lynch, J.B. (1989). Enhancement of wound healing by topical treatment with epidermal growth factor *N. Engl. J. Med.*, **321**, 76–79.

Buckley, A., Davidson, J.M., Kamerath, C.D., Wolt, T.B. and Woodward, S.C. (1985). Sustained release of epidermal growth factor accelerates wound repair. *Proc. Natl Acad. Sci. (USA).*, **82**, 7340–7344.

Buckley, A., Davidson, J.M., Kamerath, C.D. and Woodward, S.C. (1987). Epidermal growth factor increases the rate of granulation tissue development in a dose-dependent manner. *J. Surg. Res.*, **43**, 322–326.

Buckley-Sturrock, A., Woodward, S.C., Senior, R.M., Griffin, G.L., Klagsbrun, M. and Davidson, J.M. (1989). Differential stimulation of collagenase and chemotactic activity in fibroblasts derived from rat wound tissue and human skin growth factors. *J. Cell. Physiol.*, **138**, 70–78.

Clark, R.A.F. and Henson, P.M. (Eds) (1988). *The Molecular and Cellular Biology of Wound Repair*, Plenum, New York.

Davidson, J.M. and Woodward, S.C. (1989). Growth factors and wound repair: In: Abatangelo, G. and Davidson, J.M. (Eds), *Cutaneous Development, Aging, and Repair*, Liviana Press, Padova, pp. 115–139.

Davidson, J.M., Klagsbrun, M., Hill, K.E., Buckley, A., Sullivan, R., Brewer, P.S. and Woodward, S.C. (1985). Accelerated wound repair, cell proliferation, and collagen accumulation are produced by a cartilage-derived growth factor. *J. Cell Biol.*, **100**, 1219–1227.

Derynck, R. (1986). Transforming growth factor-α: structure and biological activities. *J. Cell. Biochem.*, **32**, 293–304.

Finesmith, T.H., Broadley, K.N. and Davidson, J.M. (1989). Fibroblasts from different stages of wound repair vary in ability to contract a collagen gel in response to growth factors. *J. Invest. Dermatol.*, **92**, 428a.

Grotendorst, G.R., Grotendorst, C.A. and Gilman, T. (1988). Production of growth factors (PDGF and TGF-β) at the site of tissue repair. In: Barbul, A., Pines, E., Caldwell, M. and Hunt, T.K. (Eds), *Growth Factors and Other Aspects of Wound Healing: Biological and Clinical Implications*, Alan R. Liss, New York, pp. 47–54.

McGee, G.S., Davidson, J.M., Buckley, A., Woodward, S.C., Aquino, A.M., Barbour, R. and Demetriou, A. (1988). Recombinant basic FGF accelerates wound healing. *J. Surg. Res.*, **45**, 145–153.

McGee, G.S., Broadley, K.N., Buckley, A., Aquino, A.M., Woodward, S.C., Demetriou, A.A. and Davidson, J.M. (1989). Recombinant transforming growth factor-beta accelerates incisional wound healing. *Curr. Surg.*, **46**, 103–106.

McNeil, P.L., Lakshmi, M., Warder, E. and D'Amore, P.A. (1989). Growth factors are released by mechanically wounded endothelial cells. *J. Cell Biol.*, **109**, 811–822.

Massague, J., Cheifetz, S., Ignotz, R.A. and Boyd, F.T. (1987). Multiple type-beta transforming growth factors and their receptors. *J. Cell. Physiol.*, **5**, (Suppl.) 43–47.

Montesano, R. and Orci, L. (1988). Transforming growth factor-β stimulates collagen matrix contraction by fibroblasts: Implications for wound healing. *Proc. Natl Acad. Sci. (USA)*. **85**, 4894–4897.

Mustoe, T.A., Pierce, G.F., Thomason, A., Gramates, P., Sporn, M.B. and Deuel, T.F. (1987). Accelerated healing of incisional wounds in rats induced by TGF-β. *Science*, **237**, 1333–1335.

Pierce, G.F., Mustoe, T.A., Thomas, A., Linglebach, J., Masakowski, V.R., Griffin, G.L., Senior, R.M. and Deuel, T.F. (1989). Platelet derived growth factor and transforming growth factor-β enhance tisssue repair activities by unique mechanisms. *J. Cell. Biol.*, **109**, 429–440.

Quaglino, D., Jr, Nanney, L., Ditesheim, J., Kennedy, R.Z., Broadley, K.N. and Davidson, J.M. (1989a). Localized matrix gene expression in growth factor-stimulated wound repair. *J. Cell. Biol.*, **107**, 49a.

Quaglino, D., Jr, Kennedy, R., Fornieri, C., Nanney, L., Pasquali-Ronchetti, I. and Davidson, J.M. (1989b). Matrix gene expresssion during the aging process revealed by in situ hybridization. *J. Histochem. Cytochem.*, **37**, 933.

Rapolee, D.A., Mark, D., Banda, M.J. and Werb, Z. (1988). Wound macrophages express TGFα and other growth factors *in vivo*: Analysis by mRNA phenotyping. *Science*, **241**, 708–712.

Rifkin, D.B. and Moscatelli, D. (1989). Recent developments in the cell biology of basic fibroblast growth factor. *J. Cell. Biol.*, **109**, 1–6.

Rogelj, S., Weinberg, R.A., Fanning, P. and Klagsbrun, M. (1989). Basic fibroblast growth factor fused to a signal peptide transforms cells. *Nature*, **331**, 173–175.

Sambrook, J., Fritsch, E.F. and Maniatis, T. (1989). *Molecular Cloning: A Laboratory Manual*, Cold Spring Harbor, New York.

Sato, Y. and Rifkin, D.B. (1989). Autocrine activities of basic fibroblast growth factor: regulation of endothelial cell movement, plasminogen activator synthesis, and DNA synthesis. *J. Cell. Biol.*, **107**, 1199–1205.

Sporn, M.B., Roberts, A.B., Wakefield, L.M. and deCrombrugghe, B. (1987). Some recent advances in the chemistry and biology of transforming growth factor-β. *J. Cell. Biol.*, **105**, 1039–1045.

Woodward, S.C. and Herrman, J.B. (1968). Stimulation of fibroplasia in rats by bovine cartilage powder. *Arch Surg.*, **96**, 189–199.

Wound Healing
Edited by H. Janssen, R. Rooman and J.I.S. Robertson
© 1991 Wrightson Biomedical Publishing Ltd

10

Human Keratinocyte Locomotion on Extracellular Matrix

DAVID T. WOODLEY[1], YVES SARRET[1] and EDWARD J. O'KEEFE[2]

[1]*Department of Dermatology Stanford University, California, [2]Department of
Dermatology University of North Carolina, USA*

Wound healing comprises multiple biological processes including coagulation
and formation of a fibrin clot, inflammation, re-epithelialization of the rent,
angiogenesis, wound contraction, and connective tissue repair and remodelling (Clark, 1985; 1988). Most of these processes are well-described biological
phenomena but are not understood at the cellular or biochemical level.
Although these events appear to have a precise sequence as the wound heals
(Clark, 1985; 1988), the mechanisms by which they are coordinated are not
known. Failure of any one process results in delayed healing or the formation
of a poorly healed wound.

In human beings, the most common chronic wounds are wounds of the skin
such as burns and leg or decubitus ulcers. The morbidity and mortality of
these wounds often are due to the loss of skin which exposes the patient to the
possibility of infection, metabolic changes and fluid loss. Since the skin also is
known to have immunological functions, loss of large areas of skin may
compromise the patient's immune responses. Skin has two major components, the epidermis and dermis. The epidermis is a stratified squamous
epithelium consisting largely of keratinocytes, but also of Langerhans cells,
Merkel cells and melanocytes. Langerhans cells are immunologically active
cells that process foreign antigens and communicate with the central immune
system. Melanocytes produce melanin, the primary pigment of skin which
provides protection from ultraviolet light irradiation.

Re-epithelialization could be defined as the reconstitution of all of these
cells into an organized, stratified squamous epithelium that permanently
covers the wound defect and provides the barrier properties of the skin.
However, in common parlance, re-epithelialization usually does not refer to
the reconstitution of melanocytes and Langerhans cells or even an insistence
upon a completely stratified epidermis. The wound is usually considered

re-epithelialized when the wound rent is covered by an intact epidermal membrane, the quality of which is undetermined but sufficient for keeping the moist underlying granulation tissue from appearing on the surface. It is to the advantage of the organism that the wound defect is resurfaced as quickly as possible and that a protective barrier is formed. This process must occur early after wounding and be at least partially accomplished long before the underlying connective tissue is repaired and remodelled.

In normal, unwounded skin, the keratinocyte that is juxtaposed to the basement membrane zone and the dermal connective tissue is called the *basal cell*. Within the multilayered stratified epithelium of skin, it is only the basal cell that has the potential for proliferation. In the unwounded situation, the basal cell ultimately moves off the basement membrane zone towards the surface of the skin into an area called the spinous layer or *stratum malpighian* and begins a process of 'terminal differentiation' in which the basal cell ultimately is transformed into an anucleated bag of cross-linked keratin. The stimulus for the basal cell's march toward the skin surface and the irreversible differentiation process is not known. Whether the process of terminal differentiation is signalled at the cellular level by loss of contact with the basement membrane has not been directly demonstrated.

In wound healing, the basal cells at the very margin of the wound (and those within the ablated appendage structures such as hair follicles and eccrine ducts in the wound bed) begin to behave very differently from the basal cells in unwounded skin. Their ultimate mission must be to resurface the defect, and the initial response of the cells is to migrate laterally (Stenn and Depalma, 1988) across the wound bed which consists of a fibrin and fibronectin-rich matrix (Clark *et al.*, 1982). This process usually begins within hours (Clark, 1985; 1988; Stenn and Depalma, 1988). The laterally migrating keratinocyte flattens, retracts cell–cell attachment structures (desmosomes and tonofilaments) from its plasma membrane, projects a lamellipodium and undergoes a variety of other morphological changes (Odland and Ross, 1968; Bereiter-Hahn *et al.*, 1981), but does not initiate terminal differentiation.

In consideration of the above, it appears that the basal keratinocyte behaves in two distinct modes depending upon whether it is in an unwounded or wounded environment. The mechanisms by which keratinocytes are signalled to enter the 'wound healing/migration mode' are unknown, but may include both soluble factors or extracellular matrix factors.

The extracellular matrix environment of the basal keratinocyte is very different during wound healing from that in the unwounded state. As shown in Table 1, the basal keratinocyte is juxtaposed to the cutaneous basement membrane zone in the unwounded state (Woodley *et al.*, 1985). The matrix macromolecules in this zone include the *bullous pemphigoid antigen* and *laminin*, two non-collagenous glycoproteins that are localized to the *lamina lucida zone* of the basement membrane. The lamina lucida space is

Table 1.   Keratinocyte matrices.

In unwounded state	In wounded state
Bullous pemphigoid antigen	Collagens I, III, IV, V, VI. VII
Laminin	Tenascin (hexabrachyon)
Nidogen/entactin	Fibronectin
Heparin sulphate proteoglycan	Dermatan sulphate proteoglycan
Type V collagen	Chondroitin sulphate proteoglycan
	Linkin
	Elastin
	Microfibril protein
	Fibrinogen

approximately 35 nm wide and separates the plasma membrane of the basal keratinocyte from the *lamina densa* which is a similarly sized structure in the basement membrane zone and is rich in type IV collagen. Beneath the lamina densa is a *fibrillar zone* that contains microfibrils, single collagen fibres and anchoring fibrils which contain type VII collagen (Woodley *et al.*, 1985; Sakai *et al.*, 1986). Thus, in the non-wounded situation, the plasma membrane of the basal keratinocyte rests approximately 35 nm away from the collagenous components of the basement membrane and dermis. When the skin is wounded and the basement membrane abrogated, the basal keratinocyte is no longer shielded from contact with collagens. In fact, the basal cell migrating onto the wound bed comes into contact with type IV collagen from the abrogated basement membrane, type VII collagen from anchoring fibrils and collagen types I and III in the dermis. It also comes into contact with fibrin, elastin, proteoglycans, and fibronectin, a major glycoprotein in the dermis and in the serum clot (Clark, 1985; Stenn and Depalma, 1988; Clark *et al.*, 1982; Odland and Ross, 1968; Woodley *et al.*, 1985).

Re-epithelialization involves more than locomotion since after 48–72 hours, cells at the original wound margin do proliferate and 'feed' cells in the leading edge of keratinocytes covering the wound bed (Clark, 1988; Stenn and Depalma, 1988). It is known that extracellular matrices can influence the proliferative potential and spreading of keratinocytes (Woodley *et al.*, 1990; O'Keefe *et al.*, 1985). Pure locomotion of human keratinocytes has also been demonstrated to be dramatically influenced by the matrix environment of the cell (O'Keefe *et al.*, 1985; Woodley *et al.*, 1988). Human keratinocytes are obtained from human donors and initiated into culture by the method of Rheinwald and Green (1975). The cells are subsequently passaged into serum-free MCDB 153 medium with supplements and low calcium as described by O'Keefe *et al.* (1988). This method yields predominantly monolayer cultures of keratinocytes that are in the 'basal keratinocyte state' which means that they are capable of proliferating and are not undergoing terminal differentiation. Keratinocyte cultures obtained by this method have been shown to be fibroblast-free (Petersen *et al.*, 1987). Petri dishes (35 mm) containing a glass cover-slip absorbed with albumin and gold salts were prepared as described by Albrecht–Buehler (1977). Albumin, immunoglobulin, or specific matrix molecules (collagens, fibronectin, heparin sulphate proteoglycan, or laminin) were then added to the dishes in calcium-containing Hank's balanced salt solution and allowed to immobilize on the cover-slips. Radiolabelled matrix molecules showed that approximately 60–70% of the added matrix molecule would adhere to the dish floor. Dishes were then washed and either a second matrix molecule was added and allowed to adhere or 10 000 keratinocytes suspended in 2 mm of medium were added to the dishes. Each situation was performed in triplicate. The cells were incubated for 20 hours, approximately 15 hours less than their doubling time, at 37°C in a humidified incubator with 5% CO_2 in air. The dishes were washed, fixed with formalin and viewed with dark field optics with an inverted phase microscope.

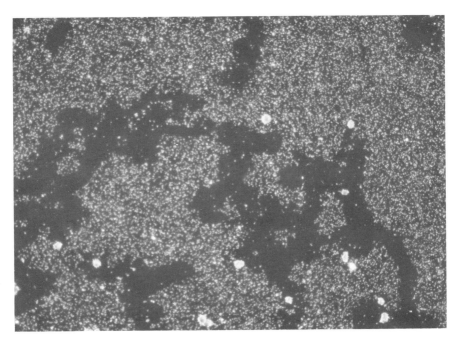

Figure 1. Human keratinocytes incubated in serum-free medium for 20 hours apposed to a type IV collagen matrix absorbed on gold salts. Note the linear black tracks formed by migrating cells that have displaced and phagocytosed the matrix and salts ($\times$ 3500).

When keratinocytes migrated during the incubation period, dark tracks were made through the gold salts due to a combination of displacement and phagocytosis (Fig. 1). The amount of locomotion was determined by photographing five random, non-overlapping fields in each dish and determining the percentage of each field occupied by locomotion tracks by the use of computer-assisted image analysis. By dividing the area of the tracks in each field by the total area of the field, a so-called *Migration index* was established for control dishes and dishes with each type of immobilized matrix. As shown in Table 2, keratinocyte locomotion was minimally influenced when the cells were in contact with cover-slips without matrix molecules or those absorbed with type V collagen, albumin or heparin sulphate proteoglycan. In contrast, fibronectin and collagen types I and IV markedly enhanced keratinocyte locomotion. Unlike all other matrices, laminin coated cover-slips inhibited keratinocyte migration. In fact, when keratinocytes were plated on a type IV collagen surface which supported migration and then laminin was added 30 min later, laminin was capable of inhibiting migration 'driven' by collagen.

Taken together, these data support the notion that laminin within the basement membrane of skin holds the basal keratinocytes in a non-migratory state. Ultrastructural studies have shown that the plasma membrane of the basal keratinocyte is apposed to laminin in normal unwounded skin (Foidart *et al.*, 1980). When the skin is injured, the cells come into contact with other basement membrane and dermal connective tissue molecules. It appears that basement membrane collagen, dermal interstitial collagen and fibronectin promote keratinocyte locomotion. Keratinocytes would come into contact with these elements during the re-epithelialization process. Other data also support this notion. Migrating keratinocytes *in vitro* and *in vivo* ultimately reconstitute the basement membrane zone when the cells have stabilized

Table 2. Keratinocyte locomotion in response to apposition with extracellular matrix components.

Matrix	Induced locomotion
Tissue culture plastic	No
Albumin	No
Immunoglobulin	No
Heparin sulphate proteoglycan	No
Type V collagen	No
Type I collagen	Yes
Type IV collagen	Yes
Fibronectin	Yes
Laminin	Inhibits locomotion

(Petersen *et al.*, 1987; Woodley *et al.*, 1980a; b; Hinter *et al.*, 1980). Both human keratinocytes and fibroblasts are capable of synthesizing laminin (Stanley *et al.*, 1982; Woodley *et al.*, 1988), and may contribute to the basement membrane zone. Laminin has a specific cell-binding domain located on the B1 chain (Timpl, 1989). This domain may communicate to the cell that it should stabilize, enter a non-migratory mode and initiate the formation of a stratified, differentiating squamous epithelium. Clark *et al.* (1982) found that in wounded guinea-pig skin laminin was not reformed in the new basement membrane zone until the keratinocytes had stopped migrating. Laminin may serve as a 'stop signal' for keratinocytes while collagens and fibronectin serve as a 'go signal' and induce the keratinocytes to migrate laterally, remain in their basal state and cover the wound.

REFERENCES

Albrecht-Buehler, G. (1977). The phagokinetic tracks of 3T3 cells. *Cell*, **11**, 395–404.

Bereiter-Hahn, J., Strohmeier, R., Kunzenbacher, I., Beck, K. and Voth, M. (1981). Locomotion of xenopus epidermis cells in primary culture. *J. Cell Sci.*, **52**, 289–311.

Clark, R.A.F. (1985). Cutaneous tissue repair: basic biologic considerations. *J. Am. Acad. Dermatol.*, **13**, 701–725.

Clark, R.A.F. (1988). Overview and general considerations of wound repair. In : Clark, R.A.F. and Hensen, P.M. (Eds), *The Molecular and Cellular Biology of Wound Repair*, Plenum Press, New York, pp. 3–33.

Clark, R.A.F., Lanigan, J.M., DellaPelle, P., Manseau, E., Dvorak, H.F. and Colvin, R.B. (1982). Fibronectin and fibrin provide a provisional matrix for epidermal cell migration during wound re-epithelialization. *J. Invest. Dermatol.*, **70**, 264–269.

Foidart, J-M., Bece, M., Yaar, M., Rennard, S.I., Gullino, M., Martin, G.R. and Katz, S.I. (1980). Distribution and immunoelectron microscopic localization of laminin, a non-collagenous basement membrane glycoprotein. *Lab. Invest.*, **42**, 336–342.

Hinter, H., Fritsch, P.O., Foidart, J.-M., Stingl, G., Schuler, G. and Katz, S.I. (1980). Expression of basement membrane zone antigens at the dermo-epibolic junction in organ culture of human skin. *J. Invest. Dermatol.*, **74**, 200–205.

Odland, G. and Ross, R. (1968). Human wound repair I. Epidermal regeneration. *J. Cell Biol.*, **39**, 135–151.

O'Keefe, E.J., Payne, R.E., Russell, N. and Woodley, D.T. (1985). Spreading and enhanced motility of human keratinocytes on fibronectin. *J. Invest. Dermatol.*, **85**, 125–130.

O'Keefe, E.J., Chiu, M.L. and Payne, R.E. (1988). Stimulation of growth of keratinocytes by basic fibroblast growth factor. *J. Invest. Dermatol.*, **90**, 767–769.

Petersen, M.J., Woodley, D.T., Stricklin, G.P. and O'Keefe, E.J. (1987). Production of collagenase by cultured human keratinocytes. *J. Biol. Chem.*, **262**, 835–840.

Rheinwald, J.G. and Green, H. (1975). Serial cultivation of strains of human epidermal keratinocytes: the formation of keratinizing colonies from single cells. *Cell*, **6**, 331–334.

Sakai, Ly, Keene, D.R., Morris, N.P. and Burgeson, R.E. (1986). Type VII collagen is a major structural component of anchoring fibrils. *J. Cell Biol.*, **103**, 1577–1586.

Stanley, J.R., Alvarez, O.M., Bere, E.W., Eaglstein, W. and Katz, S.I. (1981). Detection of basement membrane antigens during epidermal wound healing. *J. Invest. Dermatol.*, **77**, 240–243.

Stanley, J.R., Hawley-Nelson, P., Yaar, M., Martin, G.R. and Katz, S.I. (1982). Laminin and bullous pemphigoid antigen are distinct basement membrane proteins synthesized by epidermal cells. *J. Invest. Dermatol.*, **78**, 456–459.

Stenn, K.S. and Depalma, L. (1988). Re-epithelialization. In: Clark, R.A.F. and Hensen, P.M. (Eds), *The Molecular and Cellular Biology of Wound Repair*, Plenum Press, New York, pp. 321–335.

Timpl, R. (1989). Structural and biological activity of basement membrane proteins. *Eur. J. Biochem.*, **180**, 487–502.

Woodley, D.T., Regnier, M., Saurat, J. and Prunieras, M. (1980a). *In vitro* basal lamina formation may require non-epidermal living substrate. *Br.J. Dermatol.*, **103**, 397–404.

Woodley, D.T., Didierjean, L., Regnier, M., Saurat, J. and Prunieras, M. (1980b). Bullous pemphigoid antigen synthesized *in vitro* by human epidermal cells. *J. Invest. Dermatol.*, **75**, 148–151.

Woodley, D.T., O'Keefe, E.J. and Prunieras, M. (1985). Cutaneous wound healing: A model for cell-matrix interactions. *J. Am. Acad. Dermatol.*, **12**, 420–433.

Woodley, D.T., Bachman, P.M. and O'Keefe, E.J. (1988). Laminin inhibits human keratinocyte migration. *J. Cell. Physiol.*, **136**, 140–146.

Woodley, D.T., Stanley, J.R., Reese, M.J. and O'Keefe, E.J. (1988). Human dermal fibroblasts synthesize laminin. *J. Invest. Dermatol.*, **90**, 679–683.

Woodley, D.T., Wynn, K.C. and O'Keefe, E.J. (1990). Type VI collagen and fibronectin enhance human keratinocyte thymidine incorporation and spreading in the absence of soluble growth factors. *J. Invest. Dermatol.*, in press.

Wound Healing
Edited by H. Janssen, R. Rooman and J.I.S. Robertson
© 1991 Wrightson Biomedical Publishing Ltd

11

Cytoskeletal Modulation in Fibroblastic Cells in Normal and Pathological Situations

GIULIO GABBIANI

Department of Pathology, University of Geneva, CMU, Geneva, Switzerland

Mesenchymal tissues are heterogenous structures composed of cellular and extracellular elements and have multiple functional properties. Components of the extracellular matrix comprise various peptides, glycoproteins and proteoglycans that are known to fulfil essential functions in the special organization of connective tissues and to modulate the growth and differentiation of several cell types, in particular during embryonic development (Bissell *et al.*, 1982; Hay, 1981; Timpl *et al.*, 1983). Fibroblastic stromal cells, which constitute the predominant cell type in mesenchymal tissues, are responsible for the production of most connective tissue components. *In vivo*, these cells synthesize and secrete the various collagen molecules (Bornstein and Sage, 1980; Gabbiani and Rungger-Brändle, 1981). Interestingly, cultured fibroblasts synthesize different types of collagen according to their site of origin (Bernfield, 1989; Gabbiani and Rungger-Brändle, 1981).

Up to now, fibroblastic cells have been considered a relatively homogeneous population but more and more evidence is accumulating which supports the possibility that indeed fibroblasts belong to a heterogeneous family of cells and that these cells can be modulated during physiological and pathological situations. Up to now, the expression of cytoskeletal and contractile proteins has been the best marker for following these fibroblastic modulations and for relating them to different functional activities (Rungger-Brändle and Gabbiani, 1983; Sappino *et al.*, 1990; Skalli and Gabbiani, 1988). Evidence for a fibroblastic phenotypic diversity has been first suggested by the morphological differences observed between cells analyzed *in vivo* and *in vitro* (Gabbiani and Rungger-Brändle, 1981). *In vivo*, they have prominent rough endoplasmic reticulum and Golgi apparatus; their cytoplasm contains vesicles, vacuoles and numerous mitochondria. Usually, they display few microfilaments and intermediate filaments and do not establish contacts among themselves. In contrast, cultured fibroblasts show a flattened and polarized shape, possess numerous stress fibres and are interconnected by gap junctions. Cultured fibroblasts have been shown to possess the capacity of differentiating into several morphological and biochemical types which may correspond to modulations observed *in vivo* (Bayreuther *et al.*, 1988). Ultrastructural studies have confirmed that phenotypic modulations of fibroblasts occur *in vivo*. Fibroblastic cells endowed with specialized structural and functional properties have been particularly well characterized in wound repair processes (Gabbiani *et al.*, 1971; Sappino *et al.*, 1990; Skalli and Gabbiani, 1988). The initial description of these cells, or myofibroblasts, in granulation tissue was based on ultrastructural features, the most typical of which was the presence of cytoplasmic longitudinal bundles of microfilaments (stress fibres) with scattered dense bodies (Gabbiani *et al.*, 1971). Using the same criteria, myofibroblasts were described in several pathological settings related to connective tissue retraction and also in normal soft tissue (e.g. pulmonary septa) where it has been suggested they exert contractile activities (Sappino *et al.*, 1990; Skalli and Gabbiani, 1988). Granulation tissue fibroblasts have traditionally been thought to derive locally from resident cells and the observation that cultured fibroblasts show several morphologic and biochemical features of myofibroblasts is in agreement with this suggestion (Gabbiani and Rungger-Brändle, 1981). However, the possibility remains that myofibroblasts derive from local smooth muscle cells or pericytes which may also assume in certain situations morphological features of myofibro- blasts. Recent work using α-smooth muscle actin antibodies, marker of smooth muscle differentiation, has shown that during experimental wound healing, myofibroblasts gradually develop stress fibres containing α-smooth muscle actin which disappear gradually as soon as the wound closes (Darby *et al.*, 1990).

The combined evaluation of intermediate filament proteins and actin isoforms has been of great help in identifying a spectrum of fibroblastic phenotypes leading to a re-appraisal of our current definition of myofibro- blasts (Skalli *et al.*, 1989). Indeed, the cytoskeletal characterization of stromal cells present in a variety of human and experimental soft tissue specimens, known to contain myofibroblasts, has revealed the presence of four main phenotypes: (i) expressing vimentin (V-cells); (ii) co-expressing vimentin and desmin (VD-cells); (iii) co-expresssing vimentin and α-smooth muscle actin (VA-cells), and (iv) co-expresssing vimentin, desmin and α-smooth muscle actin (VAD-cells). In granulation tissue, fibroblastic cells belong, albeit temporarily, to the VA-type. At the closure of the wound, α-smooth muscle actin disappears and myofibroblasts show apoptotic changes. In contrast, hypertrophic scars contain consistently variable proportions of V- and VA-cells, and some show in addition few VAD-cells (Skalli *et al.*, 1989). In superficial fibromatoses and scleroderma lesions, cells with smooth muscle differentiation features are always present. Fibromatoses and sclerodermal lesions differ however from hypertrophic scars in that they contain usually three fibroblastic phenotypes, i.e. V-, VA-, and VAD-cells. Interestingly, the fibromatoses appear to be the only condition in which the four phenotypes, including VD-cells, are detected. These findings suggest that during chronic pathological conditions characterized by retraction, myofibroblasts assume permanently features which are observed only temporarily during normal healing processes. This phenotypic diversity may account for the different biological behaviours of these lesions. Presently, factors which influence α-smooth muscle actin expression in fibroblasts are not known. In smooth muscle cells, α-smooth muscle actin can be modulated by extracellular components such as proteoglycans and heparin (Clowes and Karnovsky, 1977), as well as by cytokines such as γ-interferon (Hansson *et al.*, 1989), heparin producing an increased expression of α-smooth muscle actin, and γ-interferon producing a decreased expression of this protein, and of its mRNA. We do not know presently whether these observations apply to fibroblastic cells, although preliminary experiments (L. Rubbia., A. Desmoulière and G. Gabbiani, unpublished observation) suggest that both actions are observed in fibroblasts. Further studies along these lines may help in clarifying the mechanisms of wound healing and fibrosis development, and may have prognostic value, for example during the evolution of hypertrophic scars, as well as therapeutic value if the actions of heparin and γ-interferon are verified *in vivo*.

REFERENCES

Bayreuther, K., Rodemann, H.P., Hommel, R., Dittmann, K., Albiez, M. and Francz, P.I. (1988). Human skin fibroblasts in vitro differentiate along a terminal cell lineage. *Proc. Natl Acad. Sci. (USA)*, **85**, 5112–5116.

Bernfield, M. (1989). Extracellular matrix. Editorial overview. *Curr. Opinion Cell. Biol.*, **1**, 953–955.

Bissell, M.J., Hall, H.G. and Parry, G. (1982). How does the extracellular matrix direct gene expression? *J. Theor. Biol.*, **99**, 31–68.

Bornstein, P. and Sage, H. (1980). Structurally distinct collagen types. *Ann. Rev. Biochem.*, **49**, 957–1003.

Clowes, A.W. and Karnovsky, M.J. (1977). Suppression by heparin of smooth muscle cell proliferation in injured arteries. *Nature (London)*, **265**, 625–626.

Clowes, A.W., Clowes, M., Kocher, O., Ropraz, P., Chaponnier, C. and Gabbiani, G. (1988). Arterial smooth muscle cells *in vivo*: relationship between actin isoform expression and mitogenesis and their modulation by heparin. *J. Cell. Biol.*, **107**, 1939–1945.

Darby, I., Skalli, O. and Gabbiani, G. (1990). α-Smooth muscle actin is temporarily expressed by myofibroblasts during experimental wound healing. *Lab. Invest.*, in press.

Gabbiani, G., Ryan, G.B. and Majno, G. (1971). Presence of modified fibroblasts in granulation tissue and their possible role in wound contraction. *Experientia*, **27**, 549–550.

Gabbiani, G. and Rungger-Brändle, E. (1981). The fibroblast. In: Glynn, L.E. (Ed.), *Handbook of Inflammation, Tissue Repair and Regeneration, Vol 3*, Elsevier/North-Holland Biomedical Press, Amsterdam, pp. 1–50.

Hansson, G.K., Hellstrand, M., Rymo, L., Rubbia, L. and Gabbiani, G. (1989). Interferon γ inhibits both proliferation and expression of differentiation-specific α-smooth muscle actin in arterial smooth muscle cells. *J. Exp. Med.*, **170**, 1595–1608.

Hay, E.D. (1981). *The Cell Biology of the Extracellular Matrix*, Plenum Press, New York.

Rungger-Brändle, E. and Gabbiani, G. (1983). The role of cytoskeletal and cytocontractile elements in pathological processes. *Am. J. Pathol.*, **110**, 359–392.

Sappino, A.P., Schürch, W. and Gabbiani, G. (1990). The differentiation repertoire of fibroblastic cells: expression of cytoskeletal proteins as marker of phenotypic modulations. *Lab. Invest.*, in press.

Skalli, O. and Gabbiani, G. (1988). The biology of the myofibroblast: relationship to wound contraction and fibrocontractive diseases. In: Clark, R.A.F. and Henson, P.M. (Eds), *The Molecular and Cellular Biology of Wound Repair*, Plenum Publishing Corporation, New York, pp. 373–402.

Skalli, O., Schürch, W., Seemayer, T., Lagacé, R., Montandon, D., Pittet, B. and Gabbiani, G. (1989). Myofibroblasts from diverse pathologic settings are heterogeneous in their content of actin isoforms and intermediate filament proteins. *Lab. Invest.*, **60**, 275–285.

Timpl, R., Engel, J. and Martin, G.R. (1983). Laminin – a multifunctional protein of basement membranes. *Trends Biochem. Sci.*, **8**, 207–209.

Wound Healing
Edited by H. Janssen, R. Rooman and J.I.S. Robertson
© 1991 Wrightson Biomedical Publishing Ltd

12

Changing Concepts in Myofibroblast Function and Control

ROSS RUDOLPH[1,2], JERRY VANDE BERG[2,3] and GLENN F. PIERCE[4]

[1]*Division of Plastic and Reconstructive Surgery, Scripps Clinic and Research Foundation, [2]UCSD La Jolla, California, [3]Core Electron Microscopy Laboratory, Veterans Administration Medical Center, La Jolla California, and [4]Department of Experimental Pathology Amgen, Inc., Thousand Oaks, California, USA*

CLINICAL WOUND CONTRACTION

Wound contraction, for which myofibroblasts are the likely motive force, is a two-edged biological sword. Either excess or insufficient wound contraction may be a clinical problem (Rudolph, 1980). The process of wound contraction teleologically is a life-saving mechanism for wound closure. An animal in the wild which is attacked by a predator and lives, yet has a large skin and soft tissue loss on its side, must have a mechanism to close that wound, else it will succumb to infection. Wound contraction serves this purpose, by pulling the intact edges of a wound together and providing efficient closure. In the clinical situation as well, wound contraction may be used to good effect. Thus, a small full-thickness burn on the thigh of an elderly patient, or a dorsally angulated tissue loss on a fingertip, may be allowed to heal by wound contraction and produce satisfactory results. Lack of effective wound contraction is a clinical problem in wounds damaged by therapeutic radiation or DNA-binding chemotherapeutic agents such as doxorubicin. Increased wound contraction would be helpful in these chronic wounds.

Yet this efficient closure mechanism may be deforming, life-threatening, or even fatal in other settings (Rudolph, 1980). An obvious example is the large burn across a joint or on the neck. As the wound heals, normal tissues are drawn together and a grotesque flexion contraction can result. Contraction around large implants in the soft tissues of the thorax, such as breast implants and cardiac pacemakers (Rudolph *et al.*, 1981), can lead to contracture of the surrounding capsule, deformity, and pain. Deeper tissues as well can undergo contraction to the detriment of the organism. Contraction in internal organs may be followed in humans by severe dysfunctional contracture, such as in rheumatic heart disease, urethral stricture, and duodenal stricture following peptic ulcer disease. The palmar fascia in Dupuytren's contracture may pull the fingers into a fixed flexion deformity requiring surgery. As a final example, the scar tissue within the cirrhotic liver undergoes contraction and may so severely restrict liver regeneration that ultimately death may occur from liver failure. In all of these pathologic conditions, myofibroblasts have been identified by electron microscopy (Guber and Rudolph, 1978). They have also been identified as expected in the contracting tissue of an open wound following burn injury or other tissue loss.

ROLES OF MYOFIBROBLASTS IN WOUND CONTRACTION

Myofibroblasts were first identified by Gabbiani, Ryan and Majno in 1971 in wound granulation tissue. These workers identified cells by electron microscopy which share the appearence of fibroblasts and smooth muscle cells. Pharmacologic testing indicated that agents which contract or relax smooth muscle have a similar effect on stretched granulation tissue containing myofibroblasts (Gabbiani et al., 1972). Finally, wound myofibroblasts stain for both actin and myosin (Gabbiani et al., 1973). On the basis of these observations, wound myofibroblasts are considered to differentiate from wound fibroblasts.

Particularly compelling evidence for the contractile function of myofibroblasts is the correlation of their life cycle with the rate of wound contraction, as studied by electron microscopy (Rudolph et al., 1977; Rudolph, 1979). While biopsies of human contracting tissues containing myofibroblasts may have a poorly defined time sequence of activity, experimental studies have been able to document the strong correlation of the myofibroblast population and active contraction. In both pigs and rats, excision of a full-thickness skin section results in a wound which has a predictable decrease in area over approximately 8 weeks in pigs (Fig. 1) and three weeks in rats (Fig. 3). During this same period, the percentage of fibroblasts within the granulating wound having myofibroblast characteristics is quite high, approaching 90% in pigs and 50% in rats. As the wound achieves its stable area after contraction, the myofibroblast population drops off (Figs. 2 and 4).

In both humans and experimental animals, full-thickness skin grafts, containing the deeper portions of the dermis, will inhibit wound contraction (Rudolph, 1979). Split-thickness skin grafts, containing epidermis and a portion of the upper dermis, will only partially inhibit wound contraction (Fig. 3). At the same time that the modification in wound contraction occurs, the myofibroblast population changes accordingly (Fig. 4). While in all types of rat wounds – open, grafted with split-thickness, or grafted with

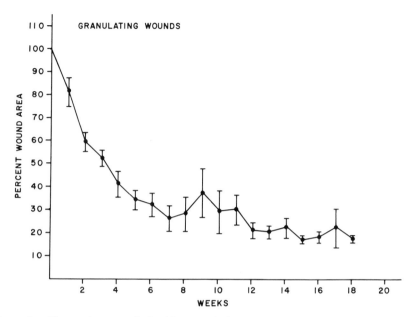

Figure 1. Change in area of pig skin granulating wounds with time. Bars indicate 1 SEM. (Reproduced with permission, from Rudolph *et al.*, 1977.)

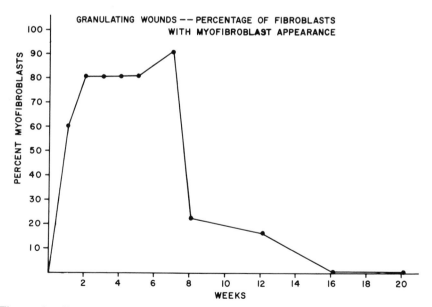

Figure 2. Percentage of fibroblasts having myofibroblast appearance in pig granulating wounds, same as Fig. 1. (Reproduced with permission, from Rudolph *et al.*, 1977.)

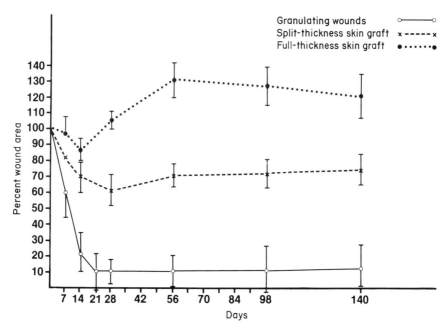

Figure 3. Change in areas of rat wounds with time. Bars indicate 1 SEM. (Reproduced with permission, from Rudolph, 1979.)

full-thickness skin grafts – the myofibroblast population rapidly peaks, in the wounds with inhibition of wound contraction by full-thickness grafts, the myofibroblast population drops off very rapidly. The intermediate inhibition of contraction by split-thickness skin grafts is paralleled by an intermediate decrease in myofibroblast population. The ungrafted wounds which contract the most also have the most prolonged myofibroblast population on electron microscopy (Rudolph, 1979).

If granulation tissue explants are placed into tissue culture and compared with normal dermal explants, distinct cell populations can be identified (Vande Berg *et al.*, 1984b). While the fibroblasts derived from normal dermis develop some characteristics of myofibroblasts, nevertheless both morphologic and growth rate differences can be identified between myofibroblast and fibroblast derived cell lines. Morphologically, cells derived from myofibroblast containing granulation tissue have larger microfilament bundles with electron dense bodies. Actin quantification reveals a higher content of actin in the myofibroblast derived cells (Vande Berg *et al.*, 1989). Furthermore, the growth rate of myofibroblast derived cell lines is slower than that of normal myofibroblasts. This has been multiply documented in myofibroblasts derived

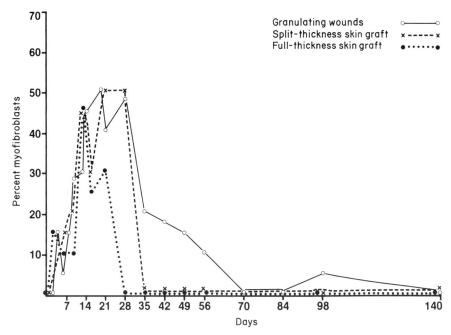

Figure 4. Observed percentage of fibroblasts having a myofibroblast appearance in the three types of rat wounds in Fig. 3. All of them developed similar numbers of myofibroblasts, but the skin-grafted wounds had a decrease in the myofibroblast population sooner. Wounds covered with full-thickness skin grafts had a more rapid decrease in myofibroblasts than did those covered with split-skin grafts. (Reproduced with permission, from Rudolph, 1979.)

from human granulation tissue (Vande Berg *et al.*, 1984b), pressure ulcers, nodules of Dupuytren's contracture (Vande Berg *et al.*, 1984a), and the contracted stroma of breast cancer (Vande Berg *et al.*, 1984c). This model of tissue culture growth curves could potentially be used to study the modulating effect of biological agents on myofibroblasts (Vande Berg and Rudolph, 1985).

Recent studies using contracted collagen gel matrices *in vitro* have questioned whether myofibroblasts are truly contractile cells or rather senescent cells. Polymerized collagen seeded with fibroblasts will undergo contraction *in vitro* in a 24–48 hour period (Bell *et al.*, 1979). During this gel contraction, the fibroblasts do not have the characteristics of myofibroblasts. Ehrlich and others (Rudolph *et al.*, 1989) have suggested from these studies that contraction of wounds is due not to intracellular contraction of myofibroblasts, but rather to fibroblasts applying tension to surrounding tissue matrix using a locomotor mechanism. Other evidence against the myofibroblast theory of wound contraction involves a number of observations. In frostbite injury, where there is minimal wound contraction, myofibroblasts are nevertheless seen (Li *et al.*, 1980). In the tight skin mouse with tissue loss, myofibroblasts peak during a time when there is no obvious wound contraction; when delayed wound contraction does occur, myofibroblasts are no longer found within the wound. These observations, and particularly the gel matrix model, have led some to suggest that myofibroblasts have no contractile function but are only senescent end-stage cells.

These studies, however, do not take into account the effect that *constant centrifugal tension* has upon *in vivo* contracting wounds, as opposed to the *in vitro* gel matrix model (Rudolph *et al.*, 1989). When a wound is made on animal or human skin, the surrounding tissue retracts. Wound contraction must close the wound against this constant outward tension. If the contracting rim is excised, the surrounding normal skin will snap back. In contrast, the contracting collagen gel model has no such outward tension, and the matrix is free to contract due to fibroblast activity with no resistance.

This point becomes important in correlating the contractile structures of myofibroblasts with structures seen in tissue cultured fibroblasts. A hallmark of the myofibroblast *in vivo* is parallel bundles of 60–80Å microfilaments containing electron-dense bodies (Rudolph, 1980). These have the same electron microscopic appearance and staining as the actin-myosin-containing contractile structures of smooth muscle cells. Fibroblasts in tissue culture develop similar bundles called 'stress filaments' if they are grown on glass or plastic plates where the cells become adherent (Burridge, 1981; Kreis and Birchmeier, 1980). It is likely that the presumably contractile bundles of myofibroblasts are homologous to these tissue-cultured, fibroblast stress filaments.

Contraction without high resistance is isotonic, whereas contraction against rigid resistance is isometric. It may well be that isotonic contraction, as in the collagen gel model, can occur without fibroblasts requiring contractile structures such as the microfilament bundles (Flesicher and Wohlfarth-Bottermann, 1975). If, however, contraction must be maintained against constant outward tension and resistance, then the larger muscle-type bundles develop within fibroblasts. Studies by Farsi and Aubin (1984) and Bellows *et al.* (1982) have shown that if a contracting collagen gel model is fixed, the fibroblasts within the gel do develop myofibroblast characteristics. If one end of the collagen gel is then released, further contraction occurs, indicating that there is still tension against resistance. Hence, myofibroblasts may play a particular role in isometric contraction, maintaining wound contraction *in vivo* against constant centrifugal tension (Rudolph *et al.*, 1989).

Regardless of whether myofibroblasts are the true motive force for contraction, it appears that at this time all investigators agree that wound contraction is an active cellular phenomenon depending on the activity of viable fibroblasts. Such cells obviously are subject to a host of biological modifiers, raising the possibility of potential control of the contraction process.

ROLES OF FIBRONECTIN AND GROWTH FACTORS IN MYOFIBROBLAST CONTROL

Current research activities in our laboratories are directed toward studying the effects of fibronectin and the growth factors transforming growth factor-β (TGF-β) and platelet-derived growth factor (PDGF) upon cultured myofibroblasts.

The influence of fibronectin on the chemotaxis of fibroblasts and myofibroblasts in tissue culture has been studied. Cells were placed in an upper chamber separated from a lower chamber by a Millipore filter (Boyden chamber) and gradients of a potential chemotaxin were placed in these chambers. The effect of increasing concentrations in both chambers, and of an increasing gradient between one chamber and the other, has become a standard method of testing for chemotaxis. Fibronectin is a protein thought to have an important role in providing a provisional matrix for fibroblasts migrating into healing wounds, and has been used clinically to increase the healing of open wounds. Fibronectin also can be seen to coat fibroblasts and myofibroblasts, and may act as an anchor for the surrounding collagen matrix.

Preliminary studies have suggested that with increasing concentrations in both upper and lower chambers, there is increased cell motility (chemo-kinesis). Using the Boyden chamber and a checkerboard analysis with varying gradients, there is a stimulatory effect on both fibroblast and myofibroblast chemotaxis in response to such gradients (Figs 5 and 6). The age of experimental animals was a factor in response. Young rat myofibroblasts has greater chemotaxis to a fibronectin gradient than did old rat myofibroblasts. Yet old rat fibroblasts demonstrated a greater chemotaxis to fibronectin gradient than did cells from young animals. We plan to continue these studies of fibronectin effect on myofibroblast activity to try to determine the effect of fibronectin on wound contraction.

Growth factors are currently receiving extraordinary attention relative to their potential effects on wound healing processes. The majority of this research has concentrated on epithelialization and on collagen synthesis in incisional wounds. Yet the healing of open and particularly chronic wounds remains a tremendous challenge, and interest is being focused on how growth factors may play a role. It has become apparent that growth factor effects on

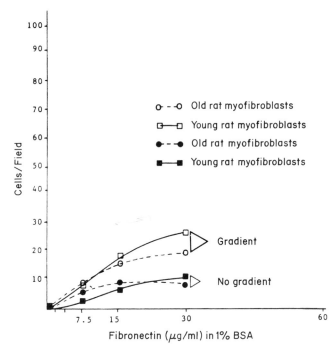

Figure 5. Dependence of young and old rat myofibroblast chemotaxis on concentration of fibronectin. Upper curves represented cells that migrated through the filter in the presence of increasing concentration of attractant in lower well. Lower curves represented random migration (chemokinesis) of cells through filter in the presence of increasing concentration of fibronectin in both upper and lower wells. Data showed that old rat myofibroblasts did not respond as well to fibronectin concentration gradient as did young rat myofibroblasts. Both populations demonstrated similar random migration. These data represent the results from five separate experiments where each value was the average of triplicate measurements. SEM did not exceed 15%.

wound healing processes are specific, i.e. stimulation of particular cellular activities in a time-dependent manner. These unique growth factors specifically influence the processes of epithelialization, angiogenesis, incisional wound healing, and open wound contraction differently.

Since wound contraction may be either beneficial or undesirable clinically, it will be essential to study the possible regulation of wound contracture by growth factors. The myofibroblast hypothesis provides an ideal model for studying growth factor activity on the wound contraction phenomenon. A few reports to date (Engrav *et al.*, 1989) have suggested that TGF-β and PDGF, the growth factors currently most studied as stimulatory agents of incisional

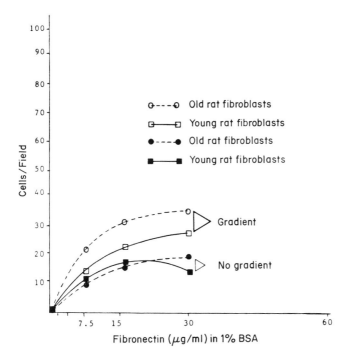

Figure 6. Dependence of old and young rat fibroblast chemotaxis on concentration of fibronectin. Experimental conditions were the same as in Fig. 5. Data showed that old and young rat fibroblasts responded chemotactically to a concentration gradient. Old rat fibroblasts appeared to respond more favourably to a fibronectin gradient than young rat fibroblasts. Both populations had a similar minimal background response when no gradient was present.

wound healing (Pierce *et al.*, 1989), do not increase the contraction rate of open wounds. These studies involved the observation and measurements of open wounds on animals' backs, and we wished to study more directly the effects of growth factors on myofibroblasts in open wounds.

An open wound model described by Mustoe *et al.* (1990) was used to study the potential influence of growth factors on myofibroblast generation in open wounds. This model involved the use of full-thickness skin excision in a rabbit ear, leaving cartilage intact. The adhesion of surrounding skin to cartilage prevents wound contraction and permits detailed analysis of the cells and new extracellular matrix within the open wound. This model has a clinical similarity to problems such as open wounds in the medial malleolus, anterior tibia or forehead, in which wound contraction is not an effective closure mechanism as surrounding tissues are unable to move freely.

In this study, purified recombinant TGF-β_1 and PDGF (BB homodimer) were applied in concentrations of 1 μg or 5 μg, respectively, to the open wounds as a single dose (Pierce *et al.*, 1990). Measurements of new granulation tissue area and volume were made at 10 and 21 days. Biopsies were taken also at 10 and 21 days and studied via light and electron microscopy. A markedly increased amount of granulation tissue was found in both the TGF-β and PDGF treated wounds at 10 and 21 days, compared with controls. Myofibroblasts were not observed in growth factor treated wounds at 10 days, but 12% of the fibroblasts were found to be myofibroblasts in the control wounds at this time. At 21 days in the PDGF and TGF-β treated wounds, less than 5% of the fibroblasts were myofibroblasts, whereas control wounds had none (Table 1). In addition, myofibroblasts from growth factor-treated, 21 day wounds did not demonstrate the marked degree of phenotypic modulation observed in control wound myofibroblasts (Figs 7 and 8). TGF-β accelerated collagen bundle formation, and PDGF accelerated glycosaminoglycan deposition, compared with control wounds, resulting in augmented granulation tissue formation and earlier closure of growth factor-treated wounds.

These data suggest an inverse relationship between the amount of new granulation tissue formed and the presence of myofibroblasts within open wounds. Thus accelerated and augmented tissue regeneration induced by PDGF or TGF-β may reduce the need for myofibroblast formation and subsequent wound contraction. In certain clinical situations it would be highly desirable to initiate growth factor stimulation of extracellular matrix deposition, collagen synthesis and epithelialization without increasing wound contraction. In large burns in particular, increased wound contraction would be an undesirable event. Thus TGF-β and PDGF may be useful in treating wounds where wound contraction is not desirable. PDGF has been shown to

Table 1.   Effect of growth factors in granulating open wounds in the rabbit ear.

	Day 10			Day 21		
	Myofibroblasts[a]	Collagen fibrils[+]	Collagen bundles[+]	Myofibroblasts[a]	Collagen fibrils	Collagen bundles
Control	+	+	−	−	+	−
TGF-β	−	+	+	+	+	+
PDGF	−	+	−	+	+	+

[a] Control wound myofibroblasts had markedly more prominent microfilament bundles and were more abundant at 10 days, compared with myofibroblasts from growth factor-treated wounds at 21 days.
+Collagen fibrils and bundles were assessed and morphometrically quantified using the Sirius Red histochemical stain and polarizing optics (Pierce *et al.*, 1990).

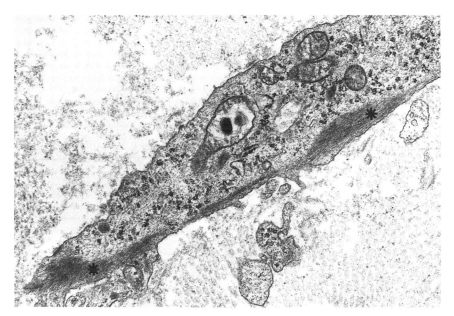

Figure 7. Myofibroblasts in 10 day control wound. The asterisks mark well-defined bundles of 60–80Å microfilaments with electron-dense bodies (× 19 500).

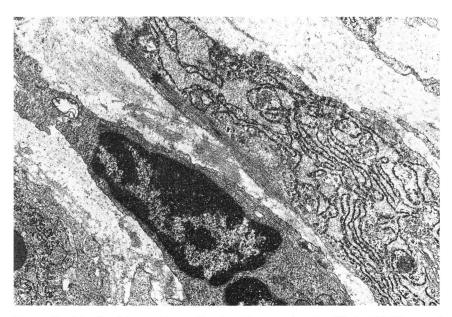

Figure 8. Myofibroblast with small microfilaments bundle (*) in PDGF-treated wound at 21 days. Microfilament bundles in growth-factor treated wounds were less developed and less prominent than in control wounds (× 14 300).

stimulate open wound re-epithelialization, likely through inductive effects, while TGF-β, a potent keratinocyte inhibitor, may inhibit re-epithelialization processes (Mustoe *et al.*, 1990).

Other polypeptide growth factors may have differing effects on wound contraction and myofibroblast generation, and may be either stimulatory or inhibitory. We plan further studies on the effect of growth factors on the wound contraction mechanism and on the induction of the myofibroblast population within wounds. The roles of TGF-β and PDGF in inhibiting differentiation of the myofibroblast phenotype may permit a more detailed examination of the role of myofibroblasts in wound contraction.

REFERENCES

Bell, E., Ivarsson, B. and Merrill, C. (1979). Production of a tissue-like structure by contraction of collagen lattices by human fibroblasts of different proliferative potential *in vivo*. *Proc. Natl Acad. Sci. (USA)*, **76**, 1274–1278.

Bellows, C.G., Melcher, A.H. and Aubin, J.E. (1982). Association between tension and orientation of periodontal ligament fibroblasts and exogenous collagen fibres in collagen gels *in vitro*. *J. Cell Sci.*, **58**, 125–138.

Burridge, K. (1981). Are stress fibers contractile? *Nature*, **294**, 691–692.

Engrav, L.H., Richey, K.J., Kao, C.C. and Murray, M.J. (1989). Topical growth factors and wound contraction in the rat: Part II, platelet-derived growth factor and wound contraction in normal and steroid-impaired rats. *Ann. Plast. Surg.*, **23**, 245–248.

Farsi, J.M.P. and Aubin, J.E. (1984). Microfilament rearrangements during fibroblast-induced contraction of three-dimensional hydrated collagen gels. *Cell Motil.*, **4**, 29–40.

Flesicher, M. and Wohlfarth-Bottermann, K.E. (1975). Correlation between tension force generation, fibrillogenesis and ultrastructure of cytoplasmic actomyosin during isometric and isotonic contractions of protoplasmic strands. *Cytobiol.*, **10**, 339–365.

Gabbiani, G., Ryan, G.B. and Majno, G. (1971). Presence of modified fibroblasts in granulation tissue and their possible role in wound contraction. *Experientia*, **27**, 549–550.

Gabbiani, G., Hirschel, B.J., Ryan, G.B. *et al.* (1972). Granulation tissue as a contractile organ: A study of structure and function. *J. Exp. Med.*, **135**, 719–734.

Gabbiani, G., Ryan, G.B., Lamelin, J.-P., *et al.* (1973). Human smooth muscle autoantibody: Its identification as antiactin antibody and a study of its binding to 'nonmuscular' cells. *Am. J. Pathol.*, **72**, 473–488.

Guber, S. and Rudolph, R. (1978). Collective review – the myofibroblast. *Surg. Gynecol. Obstet.*, **146**, 641–649.

Kreis, T.E. and Birchmeier, W. (1980). Stress fiber sarcomeres of fibroblasts are contractile. *Cell*, **22**, 555–561.

Li, A.K.C., Ehrlich, H.P., Trelstad, R.L., *et al.* (1980). Differences in healing of skin wounds caused by burn and freeze injuries. *Ann. Surg.*, **191**, 244–248.

Mustoe, T.A., Pierce, G.F., Morishima, C. and Deuel, T.F. (1990). Growth factor induced acceleration of tissue repair through direct and inductive activities in a rabbit dermal ulcer model. *J. Clin. Invest.*, in press.

Pierce, G.F., Mustoe, T.A., Lingelbach, J., Masakowski, V.R., Griffin, G.L., Senior, R.M. and Deuel, T.F. (1989). Platelet-derived growth factor and transforming growth factor-beta enhance tissue repair activities by unique mechanisms. *J. Cell. Biol.*, **109**, 429–440.

Pierce, G.F., Vande Berg, J.S., Rudolph, R., *et al.* (1990). Platelet-derived growth factor-BB and transforming growth factor-beta 1 differentially augment inflammatory and matrix assembly phases of generation: Ultrastructural and morphologic analyses. Submitted.

Rudolph, R. (1979). Inhibition of myofibroblasts by skin grafts. *Plast. Reconstr. Surg.*, **63**, 473–480.

Rudolph, R. (1980). Contraction and the control of contraction. *World J. Surg.*, **4**, 279–287.

Rudolph, R., Guber, S., Suzuki, M. and Woodward, M. (1977). The life cycle of the myofibroblast. *Surg. Gynecol. Obstet.*, **145**, 389–394.

Rudolph, R., Utley, J. and Woodward, M. (1981). Contractile fibroblasts (myofibroblasts) in a painful pacemaker pocket. *Ann. Thorac. Surg.*, **31**, 373–376.

Rudolph, R., Ehrlich, H.P. and Vande Berg, J. (1989). Wound contraction and Scar Contracture. In: Cohen, I.K., Diegelmann, R.F. and Lindblad, W.J. (Eds), *Wound Healing: Biochemical and Clinical Aspects*, W.B. Saunders, Philadelphia.

Vande Berg, J.S. and Rudolph, R. (1985). Cultured myofibroblasts: A useful model to study wound contraction and pathological contracture. *Ann. Plast. Surg.*, **14**, 111–120.

Vande Berg, J.S., Gelberman, R., Rudolph, R., *et al.* (1984a). Dupuytren's contracture: Comparative growth dynamics and morphology between cultured myofibroblasts (nodule) and fibroblasts (cord). *J. Orthop. Res.*, **2**, 247–256.

Vande Berg, J.S., Rudolph, R. and Woodward, M. (1984b). Comparative growth dynamics and morphology between cultured myofibroblasts from granulating wounds and dermal fibroblasts. *Am. J. Pathol.*, **114**, 187–200.

Vande Berg, J.S., Rudolph, R. and Woodward, M. (1984c). Growth dynamics of cultured myofibroblasts from human breast cancer and nonmalignant contracting tissues. *Plast. Reconstr. Surg.*, **73**, 605–616.

Vande Berg, J.S., Rudolph, R., Poolman, W.L. and Disharoon, D.R. (1989). Comparative growth dynamics and actin concentration between cultured human myofibroblasts from granulating wounds and dermal fibroblasts from normal skin. *Lab. Invest.*, **61**, 532–538.

Pathophysiology of Chronic Wounds

Wound Healing
Edited by H. Janssen, R. Rooman and J.I.S. Robertson
© 1991 Wrightson Biomedical Publishing Ltd

13

Chronic Wound Models Involving Dermis and Epidermis

A.C. SANK, T. SHIMA, M. CHI, R. REICH and G.R. MARTIN[1]

Laboratory of Developmental Biology and Anomalies, National Institutes of Dental Research, National Institutes of Health, Bethesda, and [1]National Institutes on Aging, Gerontology Research Center, Baltimore, Maryland, USA

While even the most severe wounds usually heal with alacrity, certain individuals including the aged, paraplegics and diabetics do not effectively repair their wounds. These wounds are extremely troublesome to the patient and even minor trauma can result in large non-healing areas. The result is that such patients require prolonged medical care for clinical wound improvement.

While it is recognized that wound healing is a coordinated activity requiring distinct populations of cells, many systems and studies have concentrated on the formation of granulation tissue, primarily with the response of fibroblasts to various compounds. For wounds to heal efficiently, keratinocytes, endothelial cells and fibroblasts respond to growth factors produced by the blood clot at the wound site (Hunt, 1988). These cells migrate and then adhere to a supportive matrix which includes collagen, laminin and fibronectin. The accumulation of this matrix is in turn regulated by synthetic and degradative pathways. For instance in the dermis, collagen type I is synthesized by fibroblasts and endothelial cells and broken down by collagenase produced by fibroblasts, keratinocytes and macrophages (Wilhelm, 1986). The balance between synthesis and degradation should determine the rate and quality of wound repair.

In our epidermal model we have focused on the importance of keratinocytes which are the predominant cell in the epidermis. These cells migrate in a directional fashion as well as proliferate to cover the open wound. Their differentiation can be induced by the addition of calcium in moderate levels in tissue culture (Hennings *et al.*, 1980; Magee *et al.*, 1987). Similarly we have found that the addition of calcium in our *in vivo* animal model results in delayed wound healing and a chronic wound, possibly relevant to human disorders.

In the dermis, wound repair has been shown to be growth factor dependent. Transforming growth factor-β (TGF-β) (Roberts *et al.*, 1985) and platelet-derived growth factor (PDGF) (Grotendorst *et al.*, 1985). increase the rate of mesodermal cell migration and proliferation (Ross *et al.*, 1986). In the dermal model described here we utilize an anti-growth factor agent, suramin, a highly sulphated organic compound developed for the treatment of parasitic disorders, but found also to inhibit the activity of certain growth factors (Fantini *et al.*, 1989). The addition of suramin to skin wounds also impairs normal repair processes.

In this chapter we show two distinct animal models of chronic wound healing. These models are characterized by different defects of matrix repair and suggest possible therapies for the treatment of chronic wounds in human clinical trials.

METHODS

We used a guinea-pig animal model to measure various *in vivo* aspects of wound healing. Our animal models consisted of three groups with 12 animals in each.

(i) The control group consisted of animals receiving two dorsal full-thickness open 2.5 cm wounds in which was placed a collagen wafer cut to the size of the wound. These collagen wafers are rapidly hydrated by the wound fluid and adhere tightly to the underlying tissue. These wounds are then covered by a transparent plastic dressing (Tegaderm, 3M, St Paul, MN) and inspected at regular intervals throughout the 3 week test period.

(ii) Calcium treated wounds were produced in animals similar to those described above except that 50 mMol $CaCl_2$ was added initially to one of the open wounds supplementary to the collagen wafer.

(iii) Suramin-treated wounds were supplemented with 1 or 10 mg/ml of the drug. All animals were housed in individual cages. The surgical operations were carried out according to a reviewed and approved NIH protocol, the animals were anaesthetized with ketamine and rompin IM (1 ml/kg for each) and four animals were sacrificed at weekly intervals from each group. Wound healing evaluations obtained from each group included the following. (a) Histology: tissue sections were stained with hematoxylin and eosin or Mason Trichrome for collagen. (b) Rate of wound contraction: pictures of wounds taken at weekly intervals with a standard 35 mm camera, 55 mm macro lens and flash at a standard distance (Figs 1 and 2). Each picture included a ruler so that wound areas could be computer digitized (Apple Macintosh, MacMeasure) to provide estimates of surface area. Results of these wound

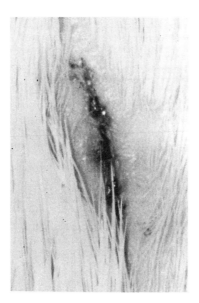

Figure 1. Normal healed wound 3 weeks after surgery. The wound has contracted down to approximately the initial wound size.

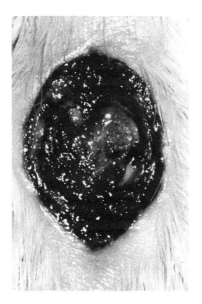

Figure 2. Calcium-treated wound at 3 weeks after surgery. The wound is large and has not contracted. Calcium delays the normal wound contraction to result in a delayed or chronic wound.

measurements are expressed as percentage wound closure with the 100% closure being the healed wound. (c) Collagen I (α_1 chain) mRNA levels (Maniatis *et al.*, 1987) were estimated by Northern hybridization on RNA isolated from the control and treated wounds (Fig. 3). Tissues obtained at the wound site were frozen at $-90°C$ until extracted with guanidine hydrochloride and sarcosyl. The extract was centrifuged over a caesium chloride gradient for 18 hours and 5 mg of the resulting RNA was electrophoresced on a denaturing agarose gel. The gel was transferred to nylon membranes and hybridized to a ^{32}P labelled probe for α_1 chain of collagen I. Filters were washed under stringent conditions, and exposed to X-ray film. The resulting bands were quantified by a densitometer. In addition, RNA from these samples were also assayed by dot blot techniques, using serial dilutions of the extracted RNA and then hybridizing the prepared filter to the labelled collagen probe. This method provides reasonable quantification of the collagen I message. (d) Collagenase assays (Wihelm *et al.*, 1986) employed a solid phase radioassay using collagen labelled with ^{125}I by the Bolton Hunter method. Tissue was homogenized in 0.15 M NaCl, 0.05 M Tris-HCl pH 7.4 at 4°C centrifuged and various amounts of the supernatant fluid were added to the wells and incubated at 37°C for 18 hours. The number of counts per well provided quantification of the collagenase activity per extracted sample. Controls consisted of buffer alone (negative control) or various amounts of fibroblast collagenase (positive control) added to wells containing labelled collagen.

These four measures were utilized to determine both the progress and underlying mechanism of the chronic wound models.

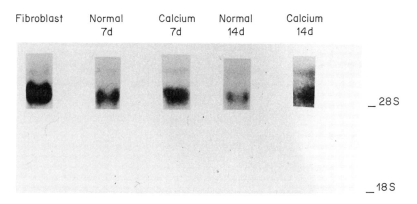

Figure 3.   Northern hybridization of RNA from normal and calcium-treated wounds to an $\alpha_1(I)$ collagen probe. This figure shows that, compared with a positive control of fibroblast mRNA, both normal and calcium treated wounds appear to express similar amounts of this gene at the time points tested.

RESULTS

Histology

The normal wounds show the anatomical detail of the three layers of the skin–epidermis, basement membrane and the dermis. In comparison, the calcium-treated model has no epithelial covering and scant collagen accumulation in the dermis. The suramin-treated wounds have very little dermal collagen visible on Mason trichrome stain.

Wound contraction

The data (Table 1) compare the rates of wound closure in normal, calcium and suramin-treated animals. The normal wounds are approximately 75% closed after 2 weeks. In contrast, the calcium-treated wounds are only 25% closed at this time and the suramin-treated group is 56% healed. The delay in contraction by $CaCl_2$ and suramin was found to be dose-dependent.

Collagen I mRNA expression

The mRNA expression (Fig. 3) was compared between the three treated groups of animals. The normal and the calcium treated groups have similar levels of mRNA for the α_1 chain of collagen I. In contrast, the suramin treated wounds show a decrease mRNA at both 2 and 3 weeks. In addition, the amount of message shown on the Northern blot decreased with increasing doses of suramin (data not shown).

Table 1.   Comparison of wound contraction in normal, suramin- and calcium-treated wounds.

Wound treatment	Wound contraction (%)
None	74 ± 6
Calcium chloride (50 mmol)	$24 \pm 6^*$
Suramin (1 mg/ml)	$56 \pm 5^*$
Suramin (10 mg/ml)	$15 \pm 4^*$

This table compares wound contraction in normal and treated wounds at 14 days after surgery. The calculation of percent wound closure is as described in the text under methodology.
* Significantly different from the control at the 0.05 level.

Table 2. Comparison of collagenase
activity in normal, suramin- and
calcium-treated wounds.

Type of wound	Collagenase activity (% normal wound)
Normal	Œ100
Calcium	124 ± 8
Suramin (1 mg/ml)	90 ± 4
Suramin (10 mg/ml)	82 ± 5

This table compares the collagenase activity
in the normal and treated wounds at 21 days
after surgery. The method of collagenase
activity is as described in the method section
in the text.
This table demonstrates the increase in
collagenase activity seen in the calcium-
treated wounds. In contrast, the suramin-
treated wounds show decreased collagenase
activity when compared with normal in
keeping with a dermal model of decreased
synthetic activity.

Collagenase activity

The three wound types are compared with regard to their individual
collagenase activity (Table 2). There is an increase in collagenase activity for
both the normal and the tested wounds to a maximum 2 weeks after surgery.
Thereafter there is a decrease in collagenase activity for both groups. The
calcium treated group has elevated collagenase activity at the time points
tested compared with either controls or suramin-treated wounds. In the
suramin-treated wounds, the collagenase activity is less than the control at all
times studied.

DISCUSSION

The data presented outline the wound healing variables seen in normal and
chronic wound models. These two models are different both in their
formulation and their matrix characterization. In the calcium supplemented
epithelial model, the keratinocytes terminally differentiate at higher
concentrations of calcium and this results in an overproduction of collagenase
which is not accompanied by changes in collagen type I gene expression. In
contrast, the suramin induced dermal model is characterized by a delay in
wound closure which is characterized by both a decrease in collagenase

activity and collagen I gene expression. We believe the calcium supplemented wounds have primarily a re-epithelialization defect while the suramin-treated wounds express a dermal defect.

Most models of chronic wounds, i.e. scurvy or lathyrism have emphasized the importance of matrix accumulation in determining the outcome of wound healing. Collagen synthesis and deposition are the principal determinants of tensile strength in the healing wound (Doillon et al., 1988). The $CaCl_2$ model emphasized the important role of degradative enzymes and suggests that the balance between synthesis and degradation is critical to normal repair and could be important to certain human lesions.

The suramin model demonstrates the importance of certain growth factors, probably PDGF and FGF, in formulating a stably healed wound. Clinically there are a number of conditions which are characterized by an overproduction of collagen, including keloids (Kelly, 1988) and hypertrophic scars. As the mechanism of suramin action involves a decrease in collagen and collagenase production, it is possible that the addition of the drug suramin to patients suffering from collagen overaccumulation could prove clinically beneficial.

These two models were established in animals. We believe that there are direct correlates between these models and clinical problems. Any interruption in the metabolism of keratinocytes would break down the metabolic barriers to the penetration of calcium into the cells and result in the terminal differentiation of keratinocytes and an epithelial defect. The dermis below such differentiated cells could be subjected to an overactivity of collagenase which would result in a degraded wound. The topical application of a calcium channel blocker, e.g. verapamil (Higgins, 1988) or a calcium chelating drug may avoid the increases of extracellular calcium which may be the initiating event in this wound model.

Chronic wounds remain a major source of patient discomfort and are a drain on resources. The creation of animal models simulating these conditions could serve to indentify possible therapeutic regimens for treating such patients. Closer investigations into the mechanisms of chronic human wounds should provide important information on the underlying defects and guide the development of new therapeutic approaches.

REFERENCES

Doillon, C.J., Dunn, M.G. and Silver, F.H. (1988). Relationship between mechanical properties and collagen structure of closed and open wounds. *J. Biochem. Eng.*, **110**, 352–356.

Fantini, J., Rognoni, J.-B., Roccabianca, M., Pommier, G. and Marvaldi, J. (1989). Suramin inhibits cell growth and glycolytic activity and triggers differentiation of human colon adenocarcinoma cell clone HT29-D4. *J. Biol. Chem.*, **264**, 10282–10286.

Grotendorst, G., Martin, G.R., Pencev, D., Sodel, J. and Harvey, A.K. (1985). Stimulation of granulation tissue formation by platelet-derived growth factor in normal and diabetic rats. *J. Clin. Invest.*, **76**, 2323–2329.

Hennings, H., Michael, D., Cheng, C., Steinert, P., Holbrook, K. and Yuspa, S. (1980). Calcium regulation of growth and differentiation of mouse epidermal cells in culture. *Cell*, **19**, 245–254.

Higgins, J.R. (1988). Angina Pectoris. In: R. Rakel (Ed.), *Conn's Current Therapy*. W.B. Saunders, Philadelphia, pp. 179–185.

Hunt, T.K. (1988). A retrospective perspective on the nature of wounds. In: Barbul, A., Pines, E., Caldwell, M. and Hunt, T.K. (Eds), *Progress in Clinical and Biological Research*, Alan R. Liss, New York, pp. xiii–xx.

Kelly, A.P. (1988). Keloids. *Dermatol. Clin.*, **6**, 413–424.

Magee, A.N., Lytton, N. and Watt, F. (1987). Calcium-induced changes in cytoskeleton and motility of cultured human keratinocytes. *Exp. Cell Res.*, **172**, 43–53.

Maniatis, T., Fritsch, E.F. and Sambrook, J. (1987). In: *Molecular Cloning. A Laboratory Manual.* Cold Spring Harbour, New York, pp. 187–211.

Roberts, A., Anzano, M.A., Wakefield, N., Roche, N.S., Stern, D.F. and Sporn M.B. (1985). Type beta transforming growth factor: A bifunctional regulator of cellular growth. *Proc Natl Acad. Sci. (USA)*, **82**, 119–123.

Ross, R., Raines, E.W. and Bowen-Pope, D.F. (1986). The biology of platelet-derived growth factor. *Cell*, **46**, 155–169.

Wilhelm, S.M., Eisen, A.Z., Teter, M., Clark, S.D., Kronberger, A. and Goldberg, G. (1986). Human fibroblast collagenase: glycosylation and tissue-specific levels of enzyme synthesis. *Proc. Natl Acad. Sci. (USA)*, **83**, 3756–3760

Wound Healing
Edited by H. Janssen, R. Rooman and J.I.S. Robertson
© 1991 Wrightson Biomedical Publishing Ltd

14

Pathophysiology of Non-healing Chronic Wounds: Biochemical Control of Grip and Stick

TERENCE J. RYAN

University of Oxford, UK

Hypertrophy and thickening of the tissues is the usual response to increased metabolic activity and is frequently a response to the injury of mechanical stress and strain (reviewed by Urschel *et al.*, 1988 and Ryan, 1989a). The forces of gravity are one determinant of differentiation (Lawless *et al.*, 1989). Lysis of tissues is the final and most complete manifestation of death. Proteolysis both within cells and outside is ever present and a requirement for living is that it should be controlled. There are several ways in which such control is determined. These include activation and inhibition or protection of the substrate either by enclosing it within a resistant membrane or coating it within materials not susceptible to lysis. Having developed such a system, nature is careful not to waste it but uses it for such phenomena as contact and adherence and even for cell recognition. Thus, antigen is susceptible to proteolysis but by protecting it by incorporation in membranes and linkage to major histocompatibility receptors, it can be preserved from lysis until immuno-surveillance has completed the recognition processes.

The observation that urokinase is co-localised with vinculin, a major constituent of the cell membrane's adhesive material (Hébert and Baker, 1988; Pollanen *et al.*, 1988) brings animal cells in line with more primitive unicellular organisms which habitually hide away a protease somewhere in their periplasm and which can be activated when lysis of the cell membrane is required for the manipulation of adherence and division of sexual activity (Buchanan *et al.*, 1989). Many cells also use activators and inhibitors of proteases for remoulding their environment, either to reshape it or to clump together within it. 'Stick' and 'grip' require that either such proteases are inhibited (Pollack and Rifkin, 1975), or that some substitute such as a glycoprotein resistant to proteases can be introduced as a locking device (Rees *et al.*, 1977). Components of the extracellular matrix determine clearance of proteases by complexing them with their inhibitors (Morton *et al.*, 1989). This is one way in which the composition of the matrix influences the remoulding of the tissues by proteolytic enzymes. Such phosphorylation is influenced by attachment and cell shape (Lee *et al.*, 1989; De Berry and Craig, 1989). The centre point for both stick and grip may well be the phosphorylation of vinculin. This requires protein kinase C to be moved from the cytoplasm and incorporated in the cell membrane (Hébert and Baker, 1988). The daunting volume of publications concerning this enzyme requires a simplified precis of its effects. The importance of protein kinase C in the transduction of biochemical signals by mechanical forces is perhaps most obvious during the development of the muscle fibre or of the myofibroblast (Adamo *et al.*, 1989); cells which function as mechanical force receptors and require phosphorylation for their response. Protein kinase C is predominantly cytosolic in mouse cultured muscle cells, but with stretch response development there is a requirement that protein kinase C should be membrane attached. Ryan (1989a) has suggested that protein kinase C is a mechanico-receptor in all cells. In the course of the development of the muscle cell there is an inverse relationship between the stretch response and the capacity to undergo mitosis (Adamo *et al.*, 1989). Several authors reviewed by Ryan (1989a) have shown that attachment, so necessary for a stretch response, is mostly incompatible with the cellular reorganization required for mitosis. When it was found that the cancer-promoting agent croton oil (PMA) activated protein kinase C and influenced cell shape and attachments, the interrelationships of many cell phenomena were clarified. Later delineation of anchorage independent growth as a feature also clarified some aspects of cell behaviour differing from the norm.

Perhaps the two most important causes of the translocation of protein kinase C to the cell membrane are calcium enrichment and mechanical distortion of the bilipid layer. Calcium effects are linked to a whole constellation of enzymes which are increasingly referred to in dermatological literature, such as calmodulin, but of equal interest is the effect of ionic binding of the phosphatides in the bilipid layer, rendering it more rigid and also increasing its electrical resistance (Nordin, 1976). These are known determinants of desmosome formation and epidermal differentiation (Mattey *et al.*, 1987). Quite as important for the transiocation of protein kinase C to the cell membrane is the depletion of the cell membrane of cholesterol (Simon *et al.*, 1989). Such depletion is a feature of desmosomes (Kitajima *et al.*, 1985). The easiest way of depleting the cell membrane is to distort it. Bending it even a little tends to push cholesterol to one side and, as a consequence, protein kinase C moves in. I have suggested that this alone justifies the concept of the transduction of biochemical signals by mechanical forces (Ryan, 1989a). There are other ways of enriching membranes with cholesterol to prevent protein kinase C moving in or depleting it to encourage the manoeuvre, but whatever the mechanism, the resulting phosphorylation processes are essential for many cell activities, including differentiation. Modifying the amount of cholesterol in the cell membrane by the distorting effects of hydrostatic forces may determine differentiation of the epidermis (Ryan, 1989a).

One environmental agent which seems to combine both chemical and mechanical effects is the glycoprotein hyaluronic acid. The chemical effect may be simply its property as a locking device for the carbohydrates on the surface of the cell (Rees et al., 1977), or conversely, the prevention of tight adhesion or the formation of hydrated pathways reviewed by Toole et al. (1989), preventing their easy slippage to one side and thus impeding the fluidity of the cell membrane. More important to physiologists and largely ignored by chemists, is the capacity of hyaluronic acid to take up water and therefore to swell, which can lead to differential mechanical forces on the cell membrane (Laurent, 1970; Toole et al., 1989). The essential effect of glycoproteins on migration, illustrated in many basic biology books (Alberts et al., 1983), is perhaps related to their capacity to influence adherence in this way. Hyaluronic acid is only one of several glycosaminoglycans now known to influence cell attachment. The mix of these may also determine swelling pressure. Hydrostatic forces are significant distorters of cell membranes and perhaps the best model for this is the endothelial cell which on one surface has to be extremely slippery and non-adhesive and on the other, has to resist the forces of flow and high blood pressure by adhering strongly. It is probably for these reasons that this cell is so well endowed with a complex adhesive versus dis-attachment system, otherwise known as coagulation and fibrinolysis and also has so many devices for resisting changes in flow or the stresses of rising blood pressure. The pathology of vascular disease includes much that is determined by haemodynamic stress. Research into atherosclerosis, aneurysms or varicose veins, includes many excursions into the study of the shape of the endothelial cell, control of its attachments and the manufacture of glycosaminoglycans or activation of proteases. Before an understanding of a weakness in the vessel wall can be realised it is necessary to know the distribution of blood flow forces and the effect of pulse (Liepsch et al., 1987; Zarins et al., 1986), the factors that determine activation of collagenase and elastase or the deposition of glycosaminoglycans (Rogers et al., 1985). The fact that endothelial cells in vivo are more elongated in regions of high shear stress (Levesque et al., 1986) needs to be interpreted in the light of in vitro studies of the same phenomenon (Eskin et al., 1989). Ryan and Barnhill (1983) suggested that such shape is likely to be correlated with more inhibition of proteolysis in order to enhance attachment, and this concept has been reviewed (Ryan, 1989a). To interpret aneurysms and varicosities one must ask whether there are sites of relatively less wall stress where cells can acquire a different shape and proteolytic enzymes are activated.

External mechanical forces are transmitted to cells via various points of attachment. Attachment and response to mechanical forces are mutually dependent. Ryan (1985; 1989a) suggested that the processes of protease inhibition are actually determined by attachment and encouraged by mechanical forces. The mechanisms include the induction of inhibitors of proteases within the cell as a direct consequence of cell membrane distortion. This is a primitive mechanism linked to actin adherence to the cell membrane and involving all the biochemistry referred to above; it underlies such phenomena as stretch receptors and depolarization, hair cells in the cochlea and their response to vibrations, or the generation of stress fibres in bone and many other phenomena correlated to mechanical stresses in wound healing. For dermatologists there are other things to think about. Scratching is perhaps the most obvious dermatological response, and widespread repetitive distortion of the skin by repetitive scratching is quite enough to explain most of the biochemical and clinical phenomena seen in atopic eczema, whether it be interleukins, phosphodiesterases or simply the release of histamine. Prurigo nodules and perhaps most pseudo-epitheliomatous hypertrophy could be a response to mechanical stresses (Grunwald *et al.*, 1988). Wound healing, skin expansion and contraction versus contracture, are other areas in which mechanical forces are induced and modify the behaviour of cells. They have been extensively reviewed but perhaps it is worth saying that skin expansion and contraction occur in all space occupying lesions including granulomata, and those which are angiocentric with palisading peripheries are ideal for the study of hydrostatic and oncotic forces on dermal behaviour. Thus, cyclical stretching of *in vitro* fibroblasts not only causes them to proliferate and to elongate but also causes them to orient themselves into concentric rings at the periphery (Mitchell *et al.*, 1989).

The effect of the mechanical forces of contracture or of expansion are to produce inhibitors of proteases such as urokinase (Masuzawa and Ryan, 1985; Masuzawa *et al.*, 1985), or of inhibitors of collagenase, as others have shown. The relationship of collagenase inhibition to shape changes of cells is well documented, as is the response to phorbol esters (Peterson *et al.*, 1989). The fact that distortion of cell membranes can have the same effect as many cytokines, including the cancer promoter PMA, has certain significant corollaries. Distorted cells respond differently to cytokines compared with cells that show no distortion. The literature includes the response to growth factors of round versus elongated cells (Gospodarowicz *et al.*, 1978) or the effect of stress on the endothelial cell on the release of prostacyclin (Frangos *et al.*, 1985; Grabowski *et al.*, 1985) or the change in ratio of heparin sulphate to chondroitin sulphate produced in response to shear stress (Mooberry *et al.*, 1989). It has also been observed that the cytokine tumour necrosis factor is effective on the neutrophil only when that cell is attached; the respiratory burst and production of oxygen-free radicals is thus determined by such attachment (Nathan *et al.*, 1989). The monocyte is stimulated to produce interleukin 1 by attachment to fibronectin (Knudsen *et al.*, 1989). Distortion of cell membranes can alter the sensitivity to signals of differentiation and is as important for abnormal behaviour, such as cancer, as any growth factor. The mechanical distortion of dermal scars has been singled out as important in promoting squamous cell epitheliomata, for instance. Important toxins like sun-induced oxygen free radicals similarly may have greater effects when the cell is in a particular shape phase, perhaps induced, for example, by the strong attachments of the facial deep wrinkle or the anatomy of the palmar fascia (Murrell *et al.*, 1987). Dupuytren's contracture is perhaps the best model of fibrosis occurring in a mild degree in almost 25% of males over the age of 65 (James, 1987), and age is the factor that I will refer to later. Dupuytren's contracture occurs at a site within the skin at which distorting forces are anatomically at a premium. Current theories about oxygen free radicals inducing this disorder (Murrell *et al.*, 1987) merely add up to the fact that any tissue undergoing stress is likely to be sensitive to toxins that act on biochemical signals which are simultaneously transduced by mechanical forces. Perhaps the most important site of stress within the skin is the epidermal–dermal junction. This at least is a province of activity by dermatologists. Ryan believes that dermatologists have ignored the fact that the papilla is a sanctuary site protected against mechanical stresses other than those induced by the hydrostatic forces of swelling pressure, whereas the rete peg is a privileged site for mechanical distortion. Similarly, the hair is a fine model for differentiation as a consequence of mechanical forces and also a model for psoriasis (Ryan, 1989a). It is perhaps worth noting Findlay's observations (1989) that hair slope is an indication of the mechanical forces subjected by the fibroblasts on those parts of the epithelium which protrude into the dermis and Rowsell's work showing that cutting the connections between the dermis and such protrusions in the embryonic rat causes instant lysis of all epithelial buds even to the extent of quite well formed whiskers (Rowsell, 1984). The papillae or the rete peg are shape changes which control stress distribution. Without such a shape, it is impossible to express either a hair or psoriasis.

There is, however, one important moderator and that is ageing. Ryan (1989a) suggests that embryonic tissues are unable to sustain inhibition of proteolysis and that adult tissues have an apparent delay in switching off such inhibitors of proteolysis (Horiuchi and Ryan, 1987). This allows the flexibility of youth to be overtaken by the fibrillogenesis and stability of ageing. I would be betraying my chief interest in blood vessels and the lymphatics as determinants of many of the controls of growth and differentiation if I did not end by pointing out that directly an organism comes of a size such that turgor alone cannot maintain skeletal function, then it is important that hydrostatic forces should be distributed. In order to control such forces, efficient sewers for the removal of effluent containing macromolecules must be designed. These are the lymphatic vessels. The fact that much of this effluent may be foreign material requiring cell recognition, ultimately links the immunological system to the lymphatics. One of the more remarkable relationships in this cell recognition system is that of the dendritic Langerhans cell within the epidermis. It is of interest that the process of immunosurveillance requires that the Langerhans cell becomes anchorage independent and finds itself speedily transported to the lymph node. One untouched area for research is how this cell is actually transported. It changes its phenotype as it migrates through the dermis (Romani *et al.*, 1989). It has been suggested that the elastin fibre is the ideal low-resistance pathway, wrapped round by materials which maintain a hydrated pathway and a coating of vitronectin with its many roles (Hintner *et al.*, 1989).

The vascular system which provides food and the lymphatic system which provides drainage is served by a remarkable cell, the endothelial cell, which on the one hand is able to control the adhesive properties of coagulation, providing a slippery surface, while at the same time maintaining firm attachments and resisting the forces of high blood pressure. The lymphatic endothelial cell is particularly spread out and unattached with its firm anchoring filaments since it has to be responsive to the external hydrostatic forces which determine much of its behaviour (Ryan, 1989b). Its mechanical sensitivity which controls the forces transmitted through the interstitium is part of the grand design of transduction of biochemical signals by mechanical forces. By something akin to a vascular system and ultimately, through its fine control, skeletal fibre deposition and removal are determined. The system which provides food and drainage should also control the size of the demand. There is a corollary that size control as organs mature will be associated with loss of flexibility and fibrillogenesis as well as impaired responses to mechanical forces, so that rises in blood pressure and eventual atrophy supervene. Breakdown in the control of permeability and drainage by the lymphatics will be followed by oedema and uninhibited proteolysis. Elephantiasis is the battle ground of these opposing trends. When lymphatics fail, proteolysis is all that is left to remove the agents which are responsible for oncotic pressure, but lipid deposition and fibrosis as well as bizarre hyperkeratosis are the indications that the system is poorly controlled (Casley-Smith and Casley-Smith, 1986). It has one other corollary – when we are dead and all hydrostatic pressures promoted by the cardiac pump come to nil, autolysis becomes an uninhibited process, thus fulfilling Hamlet's request 'O that this too too solid flesh would melt, thaw and resolve itself into a dew'.

REFERENCES

Adamo, S., Caporale, C., Nervi, C., Ceci, R. and Molinaro, M. (1989). Activity and regulation of calcium-, phospholipid-dependent protein kinase in differentiating chick myogenic cells. *J. Cell Biol.*, **108**, 153–158.

Alberts, B., Bray, D., Lewis, J., Raff, M., Roberts, K. and Watson, J.D. (1983). *Molecular Biology of the Cell*, Garland Publishing, New York.

Buchanan, M.J., Imam, S.H., Eskue, W.A. and Snell, W.J. (1989). Activation of the cell wall degrading protease, lysin, during sexual signalling in chlamydomonas: The enzyme is stored as an inactive, higher relative molecular mass precursor in the periplasm. *J. Cell Biol.*, **108**, 199–207.

Casley-Smith, J.R. and Casley-Smith, Judith R. (1986). *High Protein Oedema and the Benzo-Pyrones*, Lippincott, Sydney, Australia, pp. 536.

De Berry, C.S. and Craig, S.W. (1989). Phosphorylation of vinculin by proteinkinase C occurs in a restricted region of the molecule and is augmented by interaction with Talin. *J. Cell Biol.*, **109**, Abstr. 1475.

Eskin, S.G., Strickland, E.M. and Heath, J.P. (1989). Effects of shear stress on the migration and cell-substratum adhesion of cultured endothelial cells. *J. Cell Biol.*, **109**, Abstr. 394.

Findlay, G.H. (1989). Development of the springbok skin – colour pattern, hair slope and horn rudiments in *Antidorcas marsupialis*. *S. Afri. Tydskr. Dierk.*, **24**, 68–73.

Frangos, J.A., Eskin, S.G. and McIntyre, L.V. (1985). Flow effects on prostacyclin production by cultured human endothelial cells. *Science*, **227**, 1477–1479.

Gospodarowicz, D., Vlodavsky, I., Fielding, P. and Birdwell, C.R. (1978). The effects of epidermal and fibroblast growth factors upon cell proliferation using vascular and corneal endothelial cells as a model. In: Littlefield, J.W. and De Grouchy, D.J. (Eds), *Birth Defects*. Amsterdam: Excerpta Medica, 1978: 233–71.

Grabowski, E.F., Jaffe, E.A. and Weksler, B.B. (1985). Prostacyclin production by cultured endothelial cell monolayers exposed to step increases in shear stress. *J. Lab. Clin. Med.*, **105**, 36–43.

Grunwald, M.H., Yu-Yun Lee, J. and Ackerman, A.B. (1988). Pseudocarcinomatous hyperplasia. *Am. J. Dermatopath.*, **10**, 95–103.

Hébert, C.A. and Baker, J.B. (1988). Linkage of extracellular plasminogen activator to the fibroblast cytoskeleton colocalization of cell surface urokinase with vinculin. *J. Cell Biol.*, **106**, 1241–1247.

Hintner, H., Stanzl, U., Dahlbäck, K., Dahlbäck, B. and Breathnach, S.M. (1989). Vitronectin shows complement-independent binding to isolated keratin filament aggregates. *J. Invest. Dermatol.* **92**, 445A.

Horiuchi, Y. and Ryan, T.J. (1987). Phorbol ester stimulates urokinase-inhibitor synthesis by cultured human fibroblasts. *Br. J. Dermatol.*, **116**, 419–420.

James, J.I.P. (1987). The relationship of Dupuytren's contracture and epilepsy. *Hand*, **1**, 47.

Kitajima, Y., Sekiya, T., Moris, S., Nozawa, Y. and Yaoita, H. (1985). Freeze-fracture cytochemical study of membrane systems in human epidermis using filpin as a probe for cholesterol. *J. Invest. Dermatol.*, **84**, 149–153.

Knudsen, P.J., Linzer, R. and Dorner, M.H. (1989). Fibronectin induces transcription and accumulation of interleukin 1β RNA by U937 monocyte-like cells. *J. Cell Biol.*, **109**, Abstr. 62.

Laurent, T.C. (1970). The structure and function of the intercellular polysaccharides in connective tissue. In: Crone, C. and Lassen, N.A. (Eds), *Capillary Permeability. (Alfred Benzon Symposium II)*, Munksgaar, Copenhagen, pp. 261–277.

Lawless, B.D., Lewis, M.L., Neale, L.S. and Conda, S.R. (1989). The culture of murine bone marrow in simulated microgravity. *J. Cell Biol.*, **109**, Abstr. 1824.

Lee, S.W. and Otto, J.J. (1989). Rates of synthesis and degradation of vinculin and talin in chick fibroblasts. *J. Cell Biol.*, **109**, Abstr. 1469.

Levesque, M.J., Liepsch, D., Moravec, S. and Nerem, R.M. (1986). Correlation of endothelial cell shape and wall shear stress in a stenosed dog aorta. *Arteriosclerosis*, **6**, 220–229.

Liepsch, D.W., Steiger, H.J., Poll, A. and Reuben, H.J. (1987). Hemodynamic stress in lateral macular aneurysms. *Biorheol.*, **24**, 689–710.

Mattey, D.L., Suhrbier, Parrish, E., Garrod, D.R. (1987). Recognition, calcium and the control of desmosome formation. In: Bock, G and Clark, S (Eds), *Junctional Complexes of Epithelial Cells*, John Wiley, Chichester.

Masuzawa, M. and Ryan, T.J. (1985). Proteolysis and cell behaviour under the influence of physical force. *Int. J. Microcirc. Clin. Exp.*, **4**, 297.

Masuzawa, M., Cherry, G.W. and Ryan, T.J. (1985). Cellular proteolytic metabolism of fibroblasts and stretched skin. *Int. J. Microcirc. Clin. Exp.*, **4**, 297.

Mitchell, J.J., Absher, P.M., Baldor, L., Woodcock-Mitchell, J., Bishop, J.E., Warshaw, D., Geller, H., Hamblin, M. and Low, R.B. (1989). Mechanical strain alters cell growth and orientation of IMR-90 fibroblasts. *J. Cell Biol.*, **109**, Abstr. 1814.

Mooberry, S.L., Gardner, K.G. and Coulson, J.D. (1989). Shear stress induces modulation of endothelial proteoglycans. *J. Cell Biol.*, **109**, Abstr. 63.

Morton, P.A., Owensby, D.A. and Schwartz, A.L. (1989). Interactions between tissue-type plasminogen activator and extracellular matrix-associated plasminogen activator inhibitor-type 1 in human hepatoma cells. *J. Cell Biol.*, **109**, Abstr. 1771.

Murrell, G.A.C., Francis, M.J.O. and Bromley, L. (1987). Free radicals and Dupuytren's contracture. *Br. Med. J.*, **295**, 1373–1375.

Nathan, C., Srimal, S., Farber, C., Sanchez, E. and Kabbash, L. (1989). Cytokine-induced respiratory burst of human neutrophils: Dependence on extracellular matrix proteins and CD11/CD18 integrins. *J. Cell Biol.*, **109**, 1341–1349.

Nordin, B.E.C. (Ed) (1976). *Calcium, Phosphate and Magnesium Metabolism.* Churchill Livingstone, Edinburgh, pp. 233–234.

Peterson, M.J., Woodley, D.T., Stricklin, G.P. and O'Keefe, E.J. (1989). Constitutive production of procollagenase and tissue inhibitor of metalloproteinases by human keratinocytes in culture. *J. Invest. Dermatol.*, **92**, 156–159.

Pollack, R. and Rifkin, D. (1975). Actin-containing cables within anchorage-dependent rat embryo cells are disassociated by plasmin and trypsin. *Cell*, **6**, 495–506.

Pollanen, J., Hedman, K., Nielsen, L.S., Dano, K. and Vaheri, A. (1988). Ultrastructural localization of plasma membrane-associated urokinase-type plasminogen activator at focal contacts. *J. Cell Biol.*, **106**, 87–95.

Rees, D.A., Lloyd, C.W. and Thom, D. (1977). Control of grip and stick in cell adhesion through lateral relationships of membrane glycoproteins. *Nature*, **267**, 124–128.

Rogers, K.M., Merrilees, M.J. and Stehbens, W.E. (1985). The effect of haemodynamic stress on the glycos-aminoglycose content of blood vessel walls of experimental aneurysms and arteriovenous fistulae. *Atherosclerosis*, **58**, 139–148.

Romani, N., Lenz, A., Glassel, H., Stössel, H., Stanzl, U., Majdic, O., Fritsch, P. and Schuler, F. (1989). Cultured human Langerhans cells resemble lymphoid dendritic cells in phenotype and function. *J. Invest. Dermatol.*, **93**, 600–609.

Rowsell, A.R. (1984). The intra-uterine healing of foetal muscle wounds: experimental study in the rate. *Br. J. Plast. Surg.*, **37**, 635–642.

Ryan, T.J. (1985). The Dowling Oration: morphosis, occult forces and ectoplasm – the role of glues and proteolysis in skin disease. *Clin. Exp. Dermatol.*, **10**, 507–522.

Ryan, T.J. (1989a). Biochemical consequences of mechanical forces generated by distension and distortion. *J. Am. Acad. Dermatol.*, **21**, 115–130.

Ryan, T.J. (1989b). Structure and function of lymphatics. *J. Invest. Dermatol.*, **93**, (Suppl.) 18–24.

Ryan, T.J. and Barnhill, R.L. (1983). Physical factors and angiogenesis: In: *Development of the Vascular System (Ciba Foundation Symposium 100)*, Pitman, London; pp. 80–94.

Shirinsky, V.P., Antonov, A.S., Birukov, K.G., Sobolevsky, A.V., Romanov, Y.A., Kabaeva, N.V., Antonova, G.N. and Smirnov, V.N. (1989). Mechano-chemical control of human endothelium orientation and size. *J. Cell Biol.*, **109**, 331–339.

Simon, A.D., Steingart, R., Michel, B. and Milner, Y. (1989). Protein kinase C translocation in human and guinea-pig keratinocytes – The role of membrane physical organization (Abstract). *J. Invest. Dermatol.*, **92**, 519.

Toole, B.P., Knudson, C.B., Munaim, S.I., Knudson, W., Welles, S. and Chi-Rosso, G. (1989). Hyaluronate-cell interactions and regulation of hyaluronate synthesis during embryonic limb development. In: Abatangelo, G. and Davidson, J.M. (Eds), *Cutaneous Development, Aging and Repair.*: Fidia Research Series, Liviana Press, Padova, pp. 41–50.

Urschel, J.D., Scott, P.G. and Williams, H.T.G. (1988). The effect of mechanical stress on soft and hard tissue repair: a review. *Br. J. Plast. Surg.*, **41**, 182–186.

Zarins, C.K., Runyon-Hass, A., Zatina, M.A., Chien-Tai, L. and Glagor, S. (1986). Increased collagenase activity in early aneurysmal dilatation. *J. Vasc. Surg.*, **3**, 238–248.

Wound Healing
Edited by H. Janssen, R. Rooman and J.I.S. Robertson
© 1991 Wrightson Biomedical Publishing Ltd

15

The Human Microcirculation

JOHN E. TOOKE[1] and BENGT FAGRELL[2]

[1]*Post Graduate Medical Centre, Royal Devon and Exeter Hospital, Exeter, UK, and*
[2]*Karolinska Institute, Department of Medicine, Danderyd Hospital, Sweden*

BASIC PHYSIOLOGY AND PATHOPHYSIOLOGY

Four hundred years ago William Harvey deduced the existence of the microcirculation from careful clinical and anatomical observation (Franklin, 1963). It was many years before the existence of microchannels connecting the arteries and veins was confirmed, and only in the last 15 years have adequate tools become available through technological innovation to study the physiology of the human microcirculation directly *in vivo*. At the same time there has been a burgeoning of indirect methodologies such as laser Doppler flowmetry and transcutaneous oxygen tension measurement. In the first part of this review our knowledge of human microvascular structure and function as derived from unambiguous direct observation is summarized. In the second part the pathophysiology of the cutaneous microcirculation in relationship to skin ulceration will be considered.

SKIN CAPILLARY STRUCTURE AND DENSITY

The surface of the skin which in health continuously regenerates itself is nourished by million upon million papillary capillary loops which arise from a subpapillary arteriolar plexus (Fig. 1). The loops arise tangential to the skin surface over the vast majority of the body surface, and at the apex of the loop which may be anything from 100–500 μm from the skin surface depending on the thickness of the stratum corneum, the capillary dives back to drain into the subpapillary venous plexus. In certain skin areas there also exists an abundance of direct arteriovenous anastomoses which subserve the skin's thermoregulatory function. This in-parallel circulation is concentrated in the acral areas and when heat loss is required can convey 50 times the volume flow that is required for tissue nutrition (Burton, 1939). Clearly under these

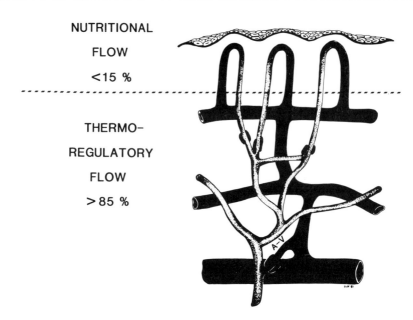

NUTRITIONAL

FLOW

<15 %

THERMO-

REGULATORY

FLOW

>85 %

Figure 1. Schematic drawing of the skin microcirculation in humans. A-V, arterio-venous anastomoses.

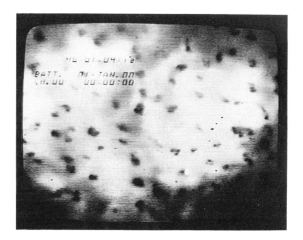

Figure 2. Photograph of the apices of capillary loops on the dorsum of the finger taken from the television screen of a television microscopy system. The area corresponds to approximately 2 mm².

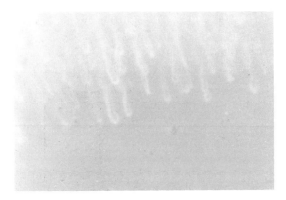

Figure 3.   Nailfold capillary loops lying parallel to the skin surface.

circumstances indirect techniques for measuring microvascular perfusion that are unable to distinguish between capillary and shunted fractions will provide a very unreliable estimate of tissue nutrition. If the skin is rendered relatively translucent by painting the surface with paraffin oil or clear varnish the apices of the capillary loops may be visualized using microscopy. Normally each dermal papilla contains between one and three such dots. Figure 2 illustrates the appearance of the skin capillaries on the dorsum of the second phalanx of the first finger visualized with a black and white television microscopy system.

In contrast, in the toe and finger nailfold the capillary loops grow parallel to the skin surface (Fig. 3). This fortuitious anatomical arrangement has permitted the majority of direct microvascular measurements to be made.

Capillary development

Direct *in vivo* microscopy studies of the skin surface of neonates suggest that the papillary loops are not formed at birth, but bud and develop to their mature form over the first few weeks of life. Microvascular structure would then appear to remain remarkably consistent, although a significant reduction in the number of visible capillary loops is evident in old age (Ryan, 1976). Study of different areas of the skin surface by television microscopy reveals marked differences in the population density of visible capillary loop apices, significantly fewer capillaries being present the further below the heart the skin is examined. The significance of this intriguing observation is unestablished, but the fact that in infancy before a child walks there appears to be little regional variation in skin capillary density, raises the possibility that hydrostatic pressure somehow determines the number of capillary loops subserving a given area of skin. It might be expected that such an adaptive response, by limiting the surface area of capillary wall available for filtration, would act to limit oedema formation in dependent parts of the body.

Amongst the other factors that are known to play a part in determining capillary density is ultra violet light, chronic exposure to which results in an atrophy of capillary loops. Much may be inferred from the structure and density of capillary loops in disease states and the ease of the technique of biomicroscopy makes it a clinically useful adjunct for assessing skin viability (*vide infra*).

CAPILLARY PRESSURE MEASUREMENT

Although the first measurements of human capillary pressure were made by Carrier and Rehberg in 1923, it was the studies of Landis in 1930 that really established the basis of our understanding of human capillary pressure control. Landis introduced glass micropipettes into the capillaries of the finger nailfold and determined the manometric pressure that needed to be applied to the pipette in order to effect no net movement of blood either into or out of the pipette tip. The capillaries were viewed using a simple microscope system (magnification × 120), the skin having been rendered translucent by painting the surface with glycerol. Positioning of the micropipette was facilitated by mounting it in a micromanipulator.

Using this system Landis was able to demonstrate that capillary pressure was higher than plasma oncotic pressure in the arterial limb of the capillary loop, but fell to values below plasma oncotic pressure in the venous limb. These observation represent the first experimental confirmation of Starling's hypothesis of transcapillary fluid balance for man, i.e. that filtration forces will tend to exceed reabsorptive forces at the arterial end of the capillary, whereas reabsorption will be favoured at the venous end. Landis also demonstrated that capillary pressure rose on local heating and fell on local cooling, and rose as the limb was lowered below the heart. In addition he showed that local histamine infiltration resulted in a rise in capillary pressure.

Much of the recent work represents a further clarification of these fundamental observations. Other workers, whilst confirming that capillary pressure is clearly higher on the arterial side of the capillary loop than the venous side, have recorded higher values for venous limb capillary pressure (Levick and Michel, 1978). In fact contemporary values tend to exceed plasma oncotic pressure, an observation that suggests a much greater reabsorptive role for post-capillary venules or the lymphatic system if tissue hydration is to remain in balance. Other workers have confirmed the positive correlation between skin temperature and capillary pressure (Fig. 4), and the increase in capillary pressure in the dependent limb. Levick and Michel (1978) however demonstrated that capillary pressure did not rise as much as

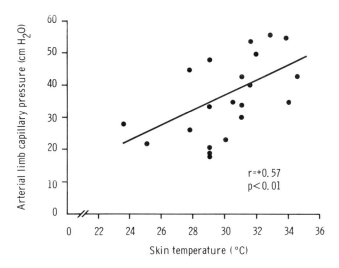

Figure 4. The relationship between nailfold capillary pressure (arterial limb of the capillary loop) and skin temperature.

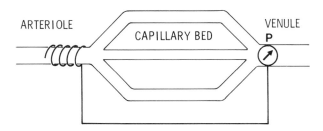

Figure 5. Diagrammatic representation of the veno-arteriolar reflex. Rise in venous pressure results in precapillary vasoconstriction, perhaps mediated by a sympathetic axon reflex, thereby limiting the rise in capillary pressure.

would be predicted from addition of the capillary pressure at heart level and the vertical distance below the heart that the extremity was placed. This important observation suggests that the ratio of pre- to post-capillary resistance rises on dependency, a response that may also be triggered by a rise in venous pressure alone, for example induced by venous occlusion. The mechanism of this response is unknown for certain, but nerve block experiments suggest that it is a sympathetic axon reflex (Hassan and Tooke, 1988), (the veno-arteriolar reflex, Fig. 5).

Alternatively it is conceivable that part of the response may depend on a myogenic mechanism, an increase in intraluminal pressure triggering vascular smooth muscle contraction (the Bayliss effect). The importance of this response relates to the prevention of oedema in circumstances in which venous pressure is raised. The resultant increase in precapillary resistance will not only limit the increment in capillary pressure, the major filtration force, but will reduce blood flow (and hence the delivery of fluid for exchange), thereby allowing haemoconcentration (and rise in plasma oncotic pressure) within the microvasulature to occur which will act as a brake to further filtration. The importance of this response as an oedema preventing mechanism in health is perhaps best illustrated by observing what happens if the response is impaired. Administration of calcium channel blockers that are potent vasodilators results in an impairment of posturally-induced vasoconstriction and consequent peripheral oedema formation not infrequently (Williams *et al.*, 1989).

In 1979 Mahler *et al.* introduced modern technology to measure capillary pressure dynamically. The principles of the technique and the merits of the method compared with manometric measurement have recently been reviewed. Briefly, a micropipette is filled with highly electrically conductive 2 M saline. On entering a capillary the saline interface is pushed into the pipette, increasing the electrical resistance across the tip which is continuously monitored. The increase in resistance results in the generation of a counter pressure that acts to restore the interface to the original position. The counter pressure (that equals capillary pressure) is recorded conventionally with a pressure transducer. The response time of this servo-nulling system is such that moment-to-moment fluctuations in capillary pressure may be discerned, including those due to cardiac pulsation (Williams *et al.*, 1988). Synchronous recording of capillary pressure, heart rate, respiration and skin blood flow has revealed other fluctuations in capillary pressure related to the respiratory cycle. The dependence of capillary pressure upon skin temperature and venous pressure has also been confirmed.

Hormonal influences on capillary pressure

By studying normal healthy women receiving a combined oral contraceptive preparation Tooke *et al.* (1981) were able to demonstrate that capillary pressure was higher in such subjects, particularly after 21 days exposure to the preparation. Compared with men, normal women studied under identical environmental conditions tend to have higher capillary pressures, but these values were approached by women on the contraceptive pill. Further evidence for the hormonal dependence of capillary pressure comes from estimates made during normal pregnancy (Tooke, 1987). Both arterial limb and venular limb capillary pressures are elevated. By the second trimester there is an increase that is sustained until term. Possible mechanisms include the increase in plasma volume that accompanies normal pregnancy (as indeed it does during contraceptive pill therapy) and/or a modulating effect of female sex hormones on peripheral vasoconstrictor mechanisms, as has been demonstrated in animal work (Altura, 1975).

CAPILLARY FLOW

The only direct method of capillary flow measurement involves recording the movement of cellular constituents of blood and plasma gaps as they pass around the capillary loop. This technique that was first described in human studies by Bollinger et al. (1974) and by Fagrell et al. (1977) may be applied to the study of capillary nailfold velocity in the finger and toe nailfold and the medial aspect of the ankle where the vessels tend to lie parallel to the skin surface. The capillaries are visualized as for pressure measurement by painting the skin surface with oil or clear varnish. The field is illuminated by a mercury vapour lamp which has an emission spectrum similar to the absorption spectrum of haemoglobin, a fact that maximizes the contrast between the intravascular red cells and the background. The image is relayed to a low light sensitivity camera and recorded on video tape for subsequent analysis. Flow velocity may either be derived by frame-to-frame analysis of the video record by recording the distance moved by plasma gaps in relation to elapsed time, or by using video photodensitometric techniques to provide a continuous read out of flow velocity. Assuming that the intra capillary red cell column is an approximation of capillary diameter and that flow is bolus in type, volume flow may be calculated from velocity and vessel radius. The disadvantage of the technique is that information from only a minute fraction of the skin capillaries may be obtained; the overriding advantage however is that the method gives an undoubted estimate of capillary flow and is not influenced by the shunt fraction. It thus represents the standard against which to judge other techniques that purport to measure capillary flow.

Characteristics of resting capillary flow

Direct recordings of nailfold capillary flow velocity support the positive correlation between skin temperature and skin blood flow suggested by nailfold capillary pressure studies and indirect methods of skin perfusion. The relationship appears to be curvilinear, flow velocity increasing steeply above a skin temperature of around 32°C (Fig. 6). The video photodensitometric technique for recording capillary flow velocity continuously has revealed characteristic fluctuations (Fig. 7) (Fagrell et al., 1977). Apart from the cardiac pulsatility that is evident in capillary flow there is a slower frequency of vasomotion that at normal skin temperatures has a frequency of about six to 10 cycles per minute. This frequency has not been related to respiration or extrinsic neural control and is thought to derive from intrinsic variation in

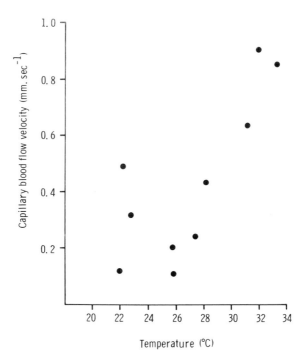

Figure 6. The relationship between nailfold capillary flow velocity and skin temperature.

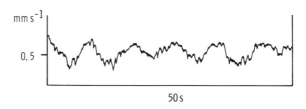

Figure 7. Vasomotion observed in human nailfold capillaries.

precapillary resistance. This view is supported by the fact that adjacent capillaries in the same field of view may be seen to be asynchronous in their flow pattern. It appears that frequency of vasomotion rises with increasing skin temperature. Vasomotion amplitude increases at first as skin temperature rises, but when maximal physiological temperatures are reached falls again as vasodilatation persists. The importance of vasomotion for the integrity of normal microvascular function is speculative, but it has been argued that such variation in pressure and flow facilitates far more efficient exchange (for a given level of volume flow rate) than continuous, steady perfusion. Furthermore, periodic increases in precapillary resistance by reducing capillary pressure allow for periods of reabsorption of fluid.

Capillary reactive hyperaemia

Study of capillary flow velocity following release of digital artery occlusion suggests that reactive hyperaemia does occur in the skin capillary bed (Tooke *et al.*, 1984), although as emphasized earlier by the digital plethysmographic studies of Patel and Burton, the degree of hyperaemia falls far short of repaying the circulatory debt incurred during the period of circulatory arrest (Burton, 1939). It has been shown by Fagrell and Östergren (1981) that the

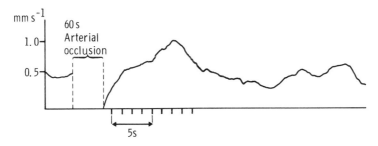

Figure 8. Post occlusive (60 s) reactive hyperaemia in a single nailfold capillary determined by videomicroscopy. The x axis refers to flow velocity in mm/s.

peak hyperaemia is reached after as little as 60 s of arterial occlusion, but the duration of hyperaemia extends with increasing occlusion duration. In health the first peak in capillary flow is reached within 5–10 s of release of occlusion, and flow returns to pre-occlusion values within one minute (Fig. 8).

The response to venous occlusion

As would be expected from capillary pressure studies, capillary flow falls by 80% or more on application of 50 mm Hg digital venous occlusion (Tooke *et al.*, 1984). A similar reduction in flow is provoked by lowering the extremity below heart level. Indeed on quiet standing toe nailfold capillary flow falls to approximately 8% of values obtained with the foot at heart level (Flynn *et al.*, 1989).

Rheological considerations

Recent years have seen a growth of interest in the rheological properties of blood. Attention has centred on *in vitro* techniques for determining blood and plasma viscosity, and for measuring blood cell deformability. The latter quantity is thought to be a particularly important determinant of blood flow through smaller vessels where vascular luminal diameter may be less than the diameter of the cell. As most of the conclusions regarding the importance of rheological factors derive from laboratory studies using bench viscometers and filtration devices to mimic conditions within the microcirculation, the *in vivo* observations of Branemark *et al.* (1971) are particularly pertinent. Branemark implanted titanium chambers in pedicle skin grafts raised on the medial aspect of the upper arm in healthy volunteers. Using this arrangement he was able to transilluminate the specimen and observe the field using high power oil immersion objectives. He described in detail cellular flow behaviour in this preparation and found no evidence of cellular occlusion of the vessels during extended periods of observation. Further insight into the *in vivo* relevance of changes in *in vitro* measures of blood rheological behaviour comes from the study of nailfold capillary flow velocity in disease states that alter blood viscosity or cell deformability (Tooke and Milligan, 1987). High blood haematocrit (polycythaemia) does not alter capillary rest flow velocity, although the achievement of peak flow after release of digital artery occlusion tends to be delayed. Studies of capillary flow velocity in patients with Waldenstrom's macroglobulinaemia in whom plasma viscosity may be grossly elevated suggests that this quantity does play a part in determining capillary flow rate, but much less than would be anticipated from *in vitro* extrapolation. Television microscopy has emphasized the potential role of the larger, much less deformable white blood cell in determining capillary flow rate. In patients with leukaemia and high leucocyte counts, capillary flow velocity was found to be very much reduced compared with values obtained after cytoreduction therapy. In addition the number of stationary capillaries approached 50% in the presence of high leucocyte counts, a finding in complete contrast to health where stationary vessels are seldom seen. In summary it is not only necessary to consider the influence of all the cellular elements of the blood, but also the capacity of the vasculature to autoregulate so as to accommodate minor increases in intrinsic resistance to flow before assuming that an *in vitro* change in viscosity results in a fall in capillary rest flow.

CAPILLARY PERMEABILITY

Capillary transfer function depends not only upon the rate of delivery of solutes for exchange but also upon the surface area and permeability of the capillary wall available for exchange. Most of our knowledge of human microvascular permeability stems from estimates of the disappearance rates of injected radiolabelled compounds, a methodology that is fraught with assumptions, and one that provides no information about the other important variables – blood flow and capillary wall area. It might thus be expected that single capillary studies would provide an important source of new information (as indeed they have in animal studies), for in the single vessel flow rate may be recorded and surface area estimated. In 1982 Bollinger *et al.* described a densitometric method for describing the diffusion patterns of sodium fluroscein around nailfold capillaries following bolus intravenous injection of the compound. By subsequently adopting a large window technique in which patterns of fluorescence were recorded from many more capillaries the method may be applied to other skin areas (Baer-Suryadinata and Bollinger, 1985).

Despite the fact that the method does not allow an estimate of true permeability (the avidity of sodium fluorescein for interstitial components is unknown for example), it has provided important new insights into capillary exchange. Of greatest interest is the observation that following intravenous injection of sodium fluorescein, the dye appears as a halo around nailfold capillary loops, suggesting that there might be a second barrier to dye diffusion placed some 10–20 μm from the capillary wall. A further important finding is that the appearance of dye is heterogeneous in time and place in cases of vascular insufficiency compared with the more or less synchronous appearance of uniformly distributed fluorescence in healthy skin. In order for us to understand more of transcapillary exchange from single vessel studies there is a need for safe, large fluorochrome-tagged molecules which thus far have not been developed.

THE MICROLYMPHATICS

The lymphatic system has for many years been the 'poor relation' of the peripheral circulation, a fact that attests to the difficulty of visualizing and measuring lymphatic function. Once more however, direct micro techniques have shed new light on the situation. Jäger and Bollinger (1985) have described the technique of fluorescence microlymphography which involves injecting with a micro-needle subepidermally 0.01 ml of fluorescein-labelled dextran. This large molecular weight compound is taken up from the interstitium by the initial lymphatics from which it has difficulty leaving in view of its large size. Using a fluorescence microscope it is possible to observe the structure and integrity of the lymphatic capillary network. In contrast to the superficial skin capillaries the normal lymph capillary network takes the form of a mesh that lies parallel to the skin surface thereafter draining into a deeper network which possesses valves.

THE MICROCIRCULATION IN DISEASE

Not infrequently the patient who develops a cutaneous wound will suffer from a disease process that exhibits characteristic microvascular changes. In peripheral arterial and venous insufficiency and diabetes mellitus the ulceration may be a direct result of the underlying disease process. The other conditions discussed here do not comprise a comprehensive list, but illustrate by way of some of the commoner diseases the manner in which microvascular structure and function might be disturbed.

Hypertension

Direct observation of the microvasculature in hypertension, for example in the retina leaves little doubt that the small vessels are influenced by the level of arterial pressure. Observers of nailfold capillaries have described in hypertension narrowing of the arterial limbs of capillary loops, widening of the venular limbs, and an increased tendency to microaneurysm formation and tortuous forms. In an analysis of microvascular organization in human conjunctiva Zweifach and coworkers found that branching patterns were disordered and microvascular rarefaction was evident in patients with established hypertension. Recently, Williams *et al.* (1986) have described capillary rarefaction in superficial skin vessels of patients with hypertension. These workers viewed the apices of capillary loops of the dermal papillae on the dorsum of the finger using television microscopy. From recorded video frames they were able to assess the number of visible capillary loops and demonstrate a reduction in capillary density that correlated with the diastolic blood pressure (Fig. 9). Reduction in capillary density in hypertension has also been demonstrated histologically for fat, cardiac and skeletal muscle (Fischer *et al.*, 1984). These observations raise important questions regarding the fixity and reversibility of the raised peripheral resistance in hypertension. In the present context the implication is that maximum microvascular perfusion might be reduced or diffusion distances increased in the skin in established hypertensives, suppositions that have clear relevance to ulcer healing and require direct experimental confirmation.

The structural changes in the cutaneous microvasculature might be taken as evidence that the capillary bed is exposed to abnormal haemodynamic influences in hypertension but the evidence for this is extremely limited in man. Eichna and Bordley studied nailfold capillary pressure in hypertensive and normotensive subjects and claimed to find no differences in resting

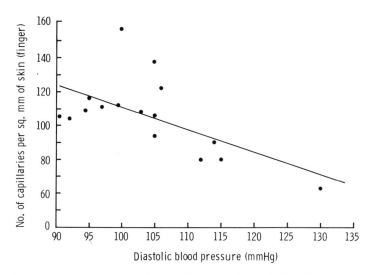

Figure 9.   Correlation between skin capillary density and diastolic blood pressure.

capillary pressure values, although re-analysis of their data suggests a tendency for capillary pressure to be higher in the hypertensive group. Following local infiltration with histamine, Eichna and Bordley (1942) did demonstrate higher pressure values in the hypertensive group demonstrating that under some circumstances at least capillary pressure may be elevated. Ostergren and coworkers studied capillary flow velocity in patients with borderline hypertension and in matched normotensive controls in response to a variety of pressor stimuli and found that the group with higher blood pressures showed a heterogeneous response with maldistribution of blood between shunt and nutritional compartments on occasion. Clearly more needs to be learnt of the microvascular haemodynamic consequences of a condition that afflicts such a large proportion of the population.

Arterial occlusive disease

Most of the studies of capillary morphology in arterial occlusive disease have been performed in the feet of patients with atherosclerosis. Fagrell (1973) visualized superficial skin capillary loops using a simple light microscope arrangement with a magnification of × 60 and incident blue light. With this system Fagrell classified skin capillaries into six stages, although for clinical purposes this may be simplified to three.

Higher stages characterized by capillary dilatation, capillary haemorrhage and sparcity of blood-filled capillaries were shown to be associated with an increased risk of subsequent skin necrosis, and indeed it appears that capillary staging is more highly predictive of necrosis of the toes than digital artery blood pressure. Schwartz *et al.* (1984) measured capillary flow velocity in the toe nailfold capillaries in patients prior to arterial reconstructive surgery and found that compared with controls of a similar age, capillary hyperaemia at rest was a feature of the atherosclerotic group. However these patients were unable to mount a normal hyperaemic response following release of a brief period of arterial occlusion at the ankle, suggesting a disturbance of microvascular autoregulation. Interestingly in relation to microsurgery there appeared to be little improvement in the first week following reconstructive surgery despite marked improvement in arterial inflow to the foot.

Heart failure

There have been few studies of microvascular haemodynamics in heart failure. That by Fahr and Ershler in 1941 established the major mechanism of peripheral oedema formation in patients with right heart failure. These authors measured finger nailfold capillary pressure and found it to be markedly elevated compared with values obtained in healthy controls, and furthermore that capillary pressure fell as oedema resolved with bed rest and salt restriction.

Diabetes mellitus

Diabetic microangiopathy probably affects all the tissues of the body and haemodynamic measurements suggest that the majority of microvascular beds demonstrate an evolving spectrum of abnormalities. Initially microvascular perfusion appears to be inappropriately raised and in the dependent foot in man (Rayman *et al.*, 1983) and in the glomerulus in animal studies (Zatz *et al.*, 1986) there is evidence of capillary hypertension. With increasing duration of diabetes a limitation of maximum microvascular perfusion becomes apparent. In the skin this may be demonstrable as a limited hyperaemic response to minor trauma, be it induced by thermal or mechanical means (Rayman *et al.*, 1986), an abnormality that appears to independent of current diabetic control. The mechanism of this limited hyperaemic response is unknown but it is conceivable that early protracted capillary hypertension might result in microvascular sclerosis, limiting vasodilatation when most required. Alternatively there may be a limitation in the release of, or response to, locally generated vasoactive mediators, a view sustained by the demonstration that substance P may be depleted in diabetic cutaneous nerves (Clements *et al.*, 1984). A third abnormality that appears to be particularly evident in patients with a long duration of diabetes is a failure of autoregulation, i.e. a failure to maintain flow in the presence of a fall in arterial pressure. This abnormality has been demonstrated for the retinal, renal and subcutaneous microcirculation (Tooke, 1986). In the latter study patients with an incapacity to maintain flow showed greater quantities of PAS staining material surrounding microvessels in skin biopsy specimens. It is conceivable therefore that build up of periluminal collagen-like material might impose structural locking on the precapillary vessels thereby restricting appropriate vasodilatation.

Finally, in the cutaneous microvascular bed there is good evidence from both direct and indirect sources that excessive arteriovenous shunting of blood occurs in diabetes, particularly in patients with peripheral neuropathy or poor diabetic control (Tooke, 1986). Not only will this tend to increase capillary pressure at the venous end of the capillary and hence the tendency to oedema formation, but also by raising skin temperature the metabolic demands of the tissue will be raised (as will the need for an increased nutritive capillary blood flow.)

Venous insufficiency

For information regarding the effects venous insufficiency, i.e. incompetent valves, it is necessary to consider changes described in the skin capillaries of the lower leg in patients with chronic venous insufficiency of the lower limb. In such patients skin capillaries may be seen to assume tortuous convoluted forms and at sites of predilection for venous ulceration capillaries are markedly reduced in number. Again presumably these changes represent adaptive responses to chronic exposure to capillary hypertension consequent upon an incompetent calf muscle pump. By using a specially cconstructed oxygen electrode through which the capillaries of the lower leg could be viewed directly with a television microscopy system, Franceck and colleagues were able to demonstrate that transcutaneous oxygen tension was predictably reduced in areas of low capillary density. By studying the interstitial diffusion and clearance of intravenously injected sodium fluoroscein the same workers have demonstrated an increased transcapillary passage of dye in the post-thrombotic limb, particularly in areas bordering on avascular zones.

CONCLUSIONS

In summary, our knowledge of human microvascular physiology is far from complete, but direct studies of capillary haemodynamics and transcapillary exchange are providing the basis for an understanding of the complexities of cutaneous microvascular physiology. Most importantly such studies have emphasized how microvascular response cannot necessarily be deduced from macrovascular measurement, and that common disease processes may have profound consequences upon microvascular structure and function. Finally, the unambiguity of direct methods of microvascular assessment provides a standard against which to judge indirect methodologies that reflect some aspect of microvascular function. New technology for assessing the microcirculation is being developed at an accelerating rate, and the investigator or health professional concerned with wound healing is obliged to grasp the principles of microvascular physiology if such developments are going to be validated and applied and interpreted intelligently.

REFERENCES

Altura, B.M. (1975) Sex and oestrogens and responsiveness of terminal arterioles to neurohypophyseal hormones and catecholamines. *J. Pharmacol. Exp. Therap.* **93**, 403–412.

Baer-Suryadinata, Ch. and Bollinger, A. (1985). Transcapillary diffusion of Na-fluorescein measured by a 'large window technique' in skin areas of the forefoot. *Int. J. Microcirc.*, **4**, 217–228.

Bollinger, A., Butti, P., Barras, J.-P., Trachsler, H. *et al.* (1974). Red blood cell velocity in nailfold capillaries of man measured by a television microscopy system. *Microvasc. Res.*, **7**, 61–72.

Bollinger, A., Frey, J., Jäger, K., Furrer, J. *et al.* (1982). Patterns of diffusion through skin capillaries in patients with long-term diabetes. *N. Eng. J. Med.*, **307**, 1305–1310.

Branemark, P.-I., Lander, L., Fagerberg, S.-E. and Breine, U. (1971) Studies in rheology of human diabetes mellitus. *Diabetologia*, **7**, 107–112.

Burton, A.C. (1939). The range and variability of the blood flow in the human fingers and the vasomotor regulation of body temperature. *Am. J. Physiol.*, **127**, 437–453.

Carrier, E.B. and Rehberg, P.B. (1923). Capillary and venous pressure in man. *Skandinav. Archiv. Physiol.*, **44**, 20–31.

Clements, R.S., Aronis, N. and Leeman, S.E. (1984). Abnormal neuronal metabolism of substance P in diabetic neuropathy. *Diabetologia*, **27**, 264A.

Eichna, L. and Bordley, J. (1942). Capillary blood pressure in man. Direct measurements in the digits of normal and hypertensive subjects during vasoconstruction and vasodilation variously induced. *J. Clin. Inves.*, **21**, 711–729.

Fagrell, B. (1973). Vital capillary microscopy. A clinical method for studying changes of the nutritional skin capillaries in legs with arteriosclerosis obliterans. *Scand. J. Clin. Lab. Invest.*, Suppl. 133.

Fagrell, B. and Ostergren J. (1981). Reactive hyperaemia response in human skin capillaries after varying occlusion duration. *Bibl. Anat.*, **20**, 692–696.

Fagrell, B., Fronek, A. and Intaglietta, A. (1977). A microscope-television system for studying flow velocity in human skin capillaries. *Am. J. Physiol.* **233**, H318–321.

Fahr, G.E. and Ershler, I. (1941). Studies of the factors concerned in edema formation; hydrostatic pressure in capillaries during edema formation in right heart failure. *Am. J. Int. Med.*, **15**, 798–810.

Fischer, P., Heimgarter, W., Hartung, E. and Henrich, H. (1984). Capillary rarefaction in different organ tissues of hypertensive patients. *Int. J. Microcirc. Clin. Exp.*, **4**, 106.

Flynn, M.D., Hassan, A.A.K. and Tooke, J.E. (1989). Effect of postural charge and thermoregulatory stress on the capillary microcirculation of the human toe. *Clin. Sci.*, **76**, 231–236.

Franklin, K.J. (Translator) (1963). *William Harvey. The Circulation of the Blood and Other Writings*. Dent, London.

Hassan, A.A.K., and Tooke, J.E. (1988). Mechanism of the postural vasoconstrictor response in the human foot. *Clin. Sci.*, **75**, 379–387.

Jäger, K. and Bollinger, A. (1985). Fluorescence microlymphography, technique and morphology. In: Bollinger, A., Partsch, H. and Wolfe, J.H.N. (Eds). *The Initial Lymphatics*. George Thieme Verlag, Stuttgart.

Landis, E.M. (1930). Microinjection studies of capillary blood pressure in human skin. *Heart*, **15**, 206–208.

Levick, J.R. and Michel, C.C. (1978). The effects of position and skin temperature on the capillary pressures in the fingers and toes. *J. Physiol.*, **214**, 97–109.

Mahler, F., Maheim, M.H., Intaglietta, M., Bollinger, A. *et al.* (1979) Blood pressure fluctuations in human nailfold capillaries. *Am. J. Physiol.*, **236**, 888–893.

Rayman, G., Williams, S., Hassan, A. and Tooke, J. E. (1983). Capillary hypertension and overperfusion in the feet of young diabetics. *Diab. Med.*, **2**, 304A, A30.

Rayman, G., Williams, S.A., Spender, P.D. *et al.* (1986). Impaired microvascular hyperaemic response to minor skin trauma in Type I Diabetes. *Br. Med. J.*, **292**, 1295–1298.

Ryan, T.J. (1976). The blood vessels of the skin. *J. Invest. Dermatol.*, **67**, 110–118.

Schwartz, R.W., Friedman, A.M., Richardson, D.R. *et al.* (1984). Capillary blood flow videodensitometry in the atherosclerotic patient. *Am. J. Vasc. Surg.*, **1**, 800–808.

Tooke, J.E. (1986). Microvascular haemodynamics in diabetes mellitus. *Clin. Sci.*, **70**, 119–125.

Tooke, J.E. (1987). The study of human capillary pressure. In: Tooke, J.E. and Sinaya, L.H. (Eds). *Clinical Investigation of the Microcirculation*, Martinus Nijhoff, Mass, USA.

Tooke, J.E. and Milligan, D.W. (1987). Capillary flow in haematological disorders: the role of the red cell, white cell and plasma viscosity. *Clin. Haemorheol.*, **7**, 311–319.

Tooke, J.E., Tindall, H. and McNilol, G.P. (1981). The influence of a combined oral contraceptive pill and menstrual cycle phase on digital microvascular haemodynamics. *Clin. Sci.*, **61**, 91–95.

Tooke, J.E., Östergren, J. and Fagrell, B. (1984). Synchronous assessment of human skin microcirculation by laser Doppler flowmetry and dynamic capillaroscopy. *Int. J. Microcirc. Clin. Exp.*, **2**, 277–284.

Williams, S.A., Tooke, J. and MacGregor, G. (1986). Rarefaction of skin capillaries in hypertension. *Clin. Sci.*, **70**, 14P.

Williams, S.A., Wasserman, S., Rawlinson, D.W., Kitney, R.I. *et al.* (1988). Dynamic measurement of human capillary blood pressure. *Clin. Sci.*, **74**, 507–512.

Williams, S.A., Rayman, G. and Tooke, J.E. (1989). Dependent oedema associated with nifedipine therapy for hypertension in diabetic patients. *Eur. J. Clin. Pharmacol.*, **37**, 333–335.

Zatz, R., Dunn, R., Meyer, T.W. *et al.* (1986). Prevention of diabetic glomerulopathy by pharmacological amelioration of glomerular capillary hypertension. *J. Clin. Invest.*, **77**, 1925–1930.

Wound Healing
Edited by H. Janssen, R. Rooman and J.I.S. Robertson
© 1991 Wrightson Biomedical Publishing Ltd

16

Measurement of Tissue Oxygen Tension in Wound Repair

FINN GOTTRUP, JUHA NIINIKOSKI[1] and THOMAS K. HUNT[2]

Department of Surgical Gastroenterology, University of Odense, Denmark,
[1]*Department of Surgery, University of Turku, Finland and* [2]*Department of Surgery, University of California, San Francisco, USA*

INTRODUCTION

Oxygen supply to tissue is vital, as 95% of the energy generated to the body normally originates from aerobic pathways, and the entire oxygen store of the body would only support resting needs for a maximum of 5 min (Kreuzer and Cain, 1985). Monitoring of tissue perfusion and maintaining oxygen supply, therefore, is of importance in all types of patients. Clinical evaluation of peripheral perfusion has been based on blood pressure, cardiac output, urine output, skin temperature and capillary return. These parameters as well as arterial and venous blood gases, however, are indirect indices of perfusion. Tissue oxygen measurements provide a direct, continuous, quantitative assessment of oxygen availability to tissue; direct relationships between wound oxygen tension and promotion of healing as well as resistance to infection have been found (Hunt, 1979; Niinikoski, 1980). Since tissue oxygen tension measurements reflect the degree to which tissue perfusion has met oxygen requirements, these measurements provide data that indicate the status of tissue perfusion.

Although the first measurement of oxygen was carried out by Lavoisier in 1779, useful methods for measurement of tissue oxygen tension and peripheral tissue perfusion in clinical practice has been slow to develop. Direct subcutaneous tissue oxygen tension measurements, however, seem capable of quantifying peripheral perfusion in dogs (Gottrup *et al.*, 1987) and man (Chang *et al.*, 1983; Jonsson *et al.*, 1987), and provide an earlier and more sensitive indicator of perfusion deficits during haemorrhage in dogs than the normal haemodynamic variables (Maxwell *et al.*, 1973; Gottrup *et al.*, 1989). In chronic indolent human wounds, tissue oxygen measurements have confirmed hypoxia, and have demonstrated elevation of wound oxygen tension with hyperbaric oxygen treatment (Sheffield, 1988).

Several techniques have been developed to measure tissue oxygen tension for research as well as clinical purposes. This chapter reviews *how* and *where* to measure tissue oxygen tension and *what methods* are most convenient for measuring tissue oxygen tension in wound healing research as well as clinical practice.

HOW CAN TISSUE OXYGEN TENSION BE MEASURED?

The ability to measure wound oxygen tension is a relatively recent development. A variety of techniques are available, each having special properties and limitations. The best proved method for measuring tissue oxygen tension (pO_2) has been polarographic electrodes, but mass spectrometry has also been successfully used. Newer techniques, especially optical methods, may also become useful in research and in clinical practice.

Polarographic electrodes

The basic polarographic principle for oxygen measurement is based on an electrode system having a noble metal (gold or platinum) as a cathode and a reference electrode of silver/silver chloride. The resulting current flow in the system is proportional to the number of oxygen molecules reduced and to the pO_2 of the solution (Fatt, 1976). The first application of oxygen polarography to mammalian tissue was performed by Davies and Brink (1942) but not before Clark in 1956 placed the cathode adjacent to the anode in an electrolyte solution behind an oxygen permeable polyethylene membrane was the problem of protein 'poisoning' of the electrode solved. This type of electrode has become the standard in the field of polarographic electrodes. Since then the electrode has been improved and has been employed in a large number of versions depending on where it has to be used. The major advantages of this technique are that it has been used for many years, that it is relatively easy to handle and that the sensors and monitor are relatively small and cheap. Major disadvantages are drift during use with need for frequent calibration, temperature dependence, sensitivity to movement, and sensitivity to certain anaesthetic agents, especially halothane.

Mass spectrometry

The basic mass spectrometer principle for oxygen measurements is gas diffusion through a permeable membrane located at the end of the probe placed in the tissue. The gas mixture is transported through a tube to the mass spectrometer, where the component gases are separated and measured quantitatively according to molecular weight. Different analysers are used for separation, e.g. magnetic, quadrapole, time of flight, and gas diffusion analysers. The advantage of this method is that it can measure several tissue gases, and the recording is very stable. The disadvantages are that the response time is long and the method consumes considerable oxygen from the tissue during the measuring procedure. Furthermore the system is heavy and expensive.

Optical fluorescence

The basic optical fluorescence principle for oxygen measurement is based on the sensitivity of certain fluorescent dyes to be quenched by oxygen. The optical sensors in this system are called *optodes*. Recently a fibreoptic sensor containing an optical fibre with a dye incorporated has been developed for measuring oxygen in blood (Baker *et al.*, 1987) and this type of optode is presently being tested for measuring subcutaneous pO_2 using a Silastic tonometer system (Baxter Technology, California). The advantages of the optical fluorescence system are: (i) no oxygen is consumed during measurement; (ii) it is not influenced by protein in the tissue; (iii) it is not sensitive to movement; and (iv) it requires less frequent calibration. Although optodes are temperature-sensitive, the instrument itself is internally compensating to eliminate this variable. The main disadvantage presently is that the system needs further development and investigations before it can be used for routine clinical work.

Other methods

Other methods for measuring tissue oxygen tension have been used or are under development. These include gas chromatography, diathermy, radioactive oxygen, magnetic resonance imaging and radioisotope imaging. None of these systems, however, is presently suitable for routine clinical use.

WHERE TO MEASURE TISSUE OXYGEN TENSION

The goal is to measure the true value of tissue oxygen tension, during all physiological and pathological conditions.

Two fundamental ways of measuring tissue oxygen tension are available: direct measurement in the tissue itself, and indirect measurement on tissue surfaces.

Direct measurement of tissue oxygen tension

This method has evolved through several forms. Tissue oxygen tension can be directly measured in implantable *wire mesh cylinders* in the fluid inside. Different types of sensors have been used. *Micro-electrodes* with 2–5 μm diameter have been used by Silver (1969) for describing the oxygen tension in rabbit ear chambers. These micro-needle-electrodes can be used for measurements where a profile of the tissue pO_2 is needed, but multiple measurements have to be made if a mean value of tissue pO_2 is wanted. In

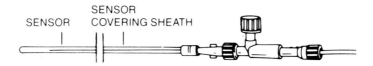

Figure 1. A coated polarographic oxygen sensor for direct placement in tissue. The catheter has a small diameter (less than 1 mm) and measures on a major area of tissue (5 mm^2).

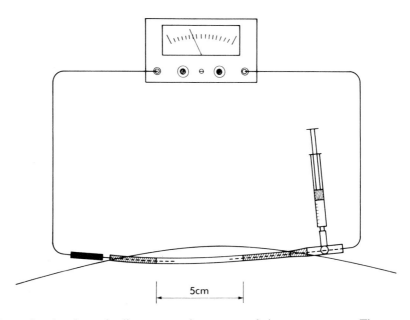

Figure 2. A schematic diagramme of one type of tissue tonometry. The oxygen needle and the three-way stopcock assembly containing the reference electrode are shown. (Reproduced with permission, from Gottrup *et al.*, 1988. © by Williams and Wilkins.)

order to measure a reproducible pO_2 of a major area of tissue the measuring area of the sensors must be much larger. Such sensors are produced both for experimental and clinical use. The sensors can be placed directly in the tissue or can measure from inside an oxygen permeable tonometer. Sensors *placed directly in tissue* must be coated in order to avoid contamination by tissue proteins. One type of coated sensor that can be placed directly in tissue is shown in Fig. 1 (Hjortdal *et al.*, 1990). The method of *tissue tonometry* is based on a single, integrated mean value of tissue pO_2 (Hunt, 1964). Different methods of oxygen tonometry have been used. Niinikoski *et al.* (1972) measured oxygen tension in human wounds by perfusing anoxic saline through the tonometer and the equilibrated saline was then measured with a standard Radiometer Clark gas monitor electrode. In a recent development of this system the pO_2 of the saline was measured in a chamber with a membrane-covered transcutaneous oxygen electrode (Larsen *et al.*, 1989). Gottrup *et al.* (1983) measured pO_2 subcutaneously using a polarographic cathode and reference placed in each end of the tube (Fig. 2). Tonometry has recently been used for subcutaneous pO_2 measurement with an optode instead of an electrode.

Indirect measurement of tissue oxygen tension

These methods are non-invasive and measure pO_2 through a tissue surface. Three types of measurements have been used experimentally as well as clinically: transcutaneous, conjunctival and transserosal.

Transcutaneous pO_2 measurement is based on a Clark polarographic electrode containing a heating element and a thermistor. The electrode must be heated to 43–44°C in order to produce measurable pO_2 values and these values will closely approximate the blood values of the dilated underlying microvessels.

In *conjunctival pO_2* and *transserosal pO_2* measurements the barrier for oxygen diffusion is only a few cell layers and there is a local temperature control. Therefore no heating is needed. Both types of sensors typically consist of a membrane-covered Clark electrode and a thermistor. In the conjunctival pO_2 system these devices are placed on a specially designed ophthalmic conformer of a material used in the manufacture of hard contact lenses (Biomedical Sensors, England) (Fig. 3). Different types of transserosal pO_2 measuring systems have been designed. Sheridan *et al.* (1987) have constructed a special system for this purpose using a small electrode directly applied by hand on the serosal surface of organs in the abdominal cavity (Fig. 4). This system has been used for prediction of colonic anastomotic healing in 50 patients. Recently Larsen *et al.* (1990) used a vacuum-fixed transcutaneous oxygen electrode on the serosal surface for measurement of oxygen tension in the gastrointestinal tract.

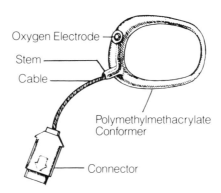

Figure 3. Conjunctival eyelid sensor for indirect measurement of oxygen tension. The conformer is placed in the eye allowing pO_2 measurement on the palpebral conjunctiva.

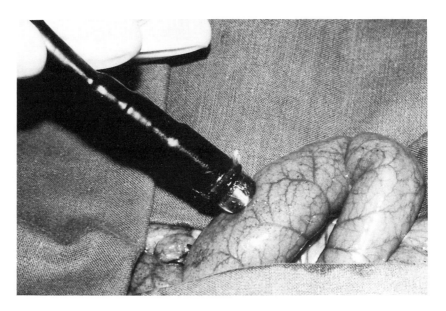

Figure 4. Transserosal sensor for indirect measurement of oxygen tension. The sensor is placed on the surface of the bowel.

What are the advantages and disadvantages of these methods?

The major disadvantage of the *directly measured oxygen tension* is that the methods are invasive. Furthermore the directly implanted non-coated electrodes may be contaminated by tissue proteins, which may alter their calibration. Coated sensors and tonometry systems do not have these difficulties and the trauma of insertion is no more than an intravenous cannula and has been well accepted by patients. More than 250 of long (Chang *et al.*, 1983) and short Silastic catheters (Gottrup *et al.*, 1983) have been inserted without experiencing problems of infection or patients' complaints for up to 2 weeks. The major advantage of the 'macro-electrode' is that it gives a direct single, integrated extracellular fluid mean value of the oxygen tension.

Indirect measuring systems have their major advantage in being non-invasive. The transcutaneous pO_2 method has been developed to measure arterial pO_2 and does so by heating the skin. The heating, however, causes major changes in local perfusion, and may induce erythema, skin blisters or burn in sensitive skin. It probably overcomes vasoconstriction, and may give a somewhat falsely optimistic value. These disadvantages are not seen using a non-heated surface pO_2 electrode. The major advantage of the conjunctival pO_2 is its insensitivity to movement while the main disadvantage is that this method cannot evaluate pO_2 of specific tissue area and that it introduces a foreign body in the eye. The transserosal pO_2 method is primarily an acute measurement because of the need for an open abdominal cavity, but it is possible to evaluate all types of tissue in the abdomen and the method is quick and easy to use.

What is measured?

What is measured by the different types of oxygen tension assays? During *normovolaemia* and changed inspiratory oxygen concentrations, transcutaneous and conjunctival oxygen tension are reliable indices of arterial tissue oxygen tension, while the directly (subcutaneously) measured pO_2 is the most useful measure of tissue oxygen (Gottrup *et al.*, 1988). During *hypovolaemia* the unheated methods of pO_2 measurements (subcutaneous and conjunctival pO_2) are reliable indicators of peripheral perfusion and tissue oxygen tension. However, the heated transcutaneous pO_2 method measures arterial pO_2 until a point is reached at which heat can no longer overcome autonomic vasoconstriction (Gottrup *et al.*, 1989). This method only assesses major perfusion deficits and is not a sensitive indicator of tissue oxygen tension under these conditions. The directly measured pO_2 is a true tissue oxygen measurement and detects changes in flow due to local vasoconstriction during all haemodynamic conditions both in experimental and human studies (Gottrup *et al.*, 1987; Ninnikoski *et al.*, 1972; Chang *et al.*,

1983; Jonsson *et al.*, 1987). The transserosal pO_2 measurement has not yet been studied as intensively as the methods mentioned above. Recent reports, however, have demonstrated a direct relationship between blood flow and mean transserosal pO_2 (Piasecki, 1985) and between pO_2 measured directly in the tissue and on its surface (Larsen *et al.*, 1990).

WHAT METHOD TO USE FOR MEASURING TISSUE OXYGEN TENSION IN WOUND HEALING RESEARCH AS WELL AS IN CLINICAL PRACTICE?

Proliferation of epithelium and of fibroblasts is to a large extent dependent on the oxygen micro-environment. This has been concluded after environmental studies describing tissue oxygen tension profiles of artificial wounds (Silver, 1969). In these types of studies *micro-electrode technique* is the best method. However, if pO_2 of a major tissue area or volume is needed other methods must be used. For these types of measurements *tissue tonometry* was used at first in minor human subcutaneous wounds (Niinikoski *et al.*, 1972). Later it was demonstrated that oxygen tension in small subcutaneous wounds in the arm varies in the same manner as oxygen tension in an operative incision. Tissue oxygen tension in the operative incision is usually lower than in the needle wound in the arm, but pO_2 of an arm wound seems to monitor the efficiency of oxygen delivery to the operative wound (Goodson *et al.*, 1984). Tissue tonometry and *transcutaneous pO_2 measurements* have shown low oxygen values of problem wounds (Sheffield, 1988). In this case the non-heated and heated electrodes read alike, probably because the perfusion is so low that heat does not influence blood flow. Nevertheless, transcutaneous pO_2 measurements in ischaemic wounds are difficult to interpret. The best data are probably offered by measuring the effects of added oxygen and posture changes. *Conjunctival pO_2 measurements* have been proven useful for evaluating haemodynamic alterations of the body and are correlated with changes in tissue oxygen tension in the subcutis. However this approach is less useful when investigating local perfusion in wound healing research. *Transserosal pO_2 measurements* have been of value in the prediction of healing of bowel anastomoses and leakage. The method is easy to use, fast and does not require special skills for interpretation of the data. This measurement may become a valuable tool in wound healing research experimentally as well as clinically.

SUMMARY

Tissue oxygen tension measurements provide an important tool for evaluating perfusion of peripheral tissues. Tissue oxygen monitoring seems to have fundamental value in prediction of wound healing and wound infection, and may be a valuable adjunct in clinical decision making in problem wounds.

REFERENCES

Baker, S.J., Tremper, K.K., Hyatt, J., Heitzmann, H.A., Holman, B.M., Pike, K., Ring, L.S., Teope, M. and Thaure, T.B. (1987). Continuous fiberoptic arterial oxygen tension measurements in dogs. *J. Clin. Monit.*, **3**, 48–52.

Chang, N., Goodson, W.H., Gottrup, F. and Hunt, T.K. (1983). Direct measurement of wound and tissue oxygen tension in postoperative patients. *Ann. Surg.*, **197**, 470–478.

Clark, L.C. (1956). Monitor and control of blood and tissue oxygen tension. *Trans. Am. Soc. Artif. Intern. Org.*, **2**, 41–46.

Davies, P.W. and Brink, F. (1942). Microelectrodes for measuring local oxygen tension in animal tissues. *Rev. Sci. Instr.*, **13**, 524–533.

Fatt, I. (1976). *Polarographic Oxygen Sensors. Its Theory of Operation and its Application in Biology, Medicine and Technology*, CRC Press, Cleveland.

Goodson, W.H. Hunt, T.K., Gottrup, F., Jonsson, K., Chang, N., Firmin, R. and West, J.M. (1984). Measurement of human repair: An overview. In: Hunt, T.K., Heppenstall, R.B., Pines, E. and Rovee, D. (Eds), *Soft and Hard Tissue Repair*, Praeger, New York, pp. 574–585.

Gottrup, F., Firmin, R., Chang, N., Goodson, W.H. and Hunt, T.K. (1983). Continuous direct tissue oxygen tension measurement by a new method using an implantable Silastic tonometer and oxygen polarography. *Am. J. Surg.*, **146**, 399–403.

Gottrup, F., Firmin, R., Rabkin, J., Halliday, B.J. and Hunt, T.K. (1987). Directly measured tissue oxygen tension and arterial oxygen tension assess tissue perfusion. *Crit. Care Med.*, **15**, 1030–1036.

Gottrup, F., Gellett, S., Kirkegaard, L., Hansen, E.S. and Johansen, G. (1988). Continuous monitoring of tissue oxygen tension during hyperoxia and hypoxia: Relation of subcutaneous, transcutaneous and conjunctival oxygen tension to haemodynamic variables. *Crit. Care Med.*, **16**, 1229–1234.

Gottrup, F., Gellett, S., Kirkegaard, L., Hansen, E.S. and Johansen, G. (1989). Effect of haemorrhage and resuscitation on subcutaneous, conjunctival and transcutaneous oxygen tension in relation to hemodynamic variables. *Crit. Care Med.*, **17**, 904–907.

Hjortdal, V.E., Timmenga, E.J., Kjølseth, D., Henriksen, T.B., Hansen, E.S., Djuurhus, J.C. and Gottrup, F. (1990). Continuous direct tissue oxygen tension measurement. A new application for an intravascular oxygen sensor. *Ann. Chir. Gynaecol.*, in press.

Hunt, T.K. (1964). A new method of determining tissue oxygen tension. *Lancet*, **ii**, 1370–1371.

Hunt, T.K. (1979). Disorders of repair and their management. In: Hunt, T.K. and Dunphy, J.E. (Eds), *Fundamentals of Wound Management*, Appleton-Century-Crofts, New York, pp. 68–168.

Jonsson, K., Jensen, J.A., Goodson, W.H., West, J.M. and Hunt, T.K. (1987). Assessment of perfusion in postoperative patients using tissue oxygen measurements. *Br. J. Surg.*, **74**, 263–267.

Kreuzer, F. and Cain, S.M. (1985). Regulation of the peripheral vasculature and tissue oxygenation in health and disease. *Crit. Care Clin.*, **1**, 453–470.

Larsen, P.N., Moesgaard, F., Gottrup, F. and Helledie, N. (1989). Characterization of the silicone tonometer using a membrane-covered transcutaneous electrode. *Scand. J. Clin. Lab. Invest.*, **49**, 513–519.

Larsen, P.N., Moesgaard, F., Naver, L., Rosenberg, J., Gottrup, F., Kirkegaard, P. and Helledie, N. (1990). Gastric and colonic oxygen tension measured by a vacuum fixated oxygen electrode. *Scand. J. Gastroenterol.*, in press.

Maxwell, T.M., Lim, R.C., Fuchs, R. and Hunt, T.K. (1973). Continuous monitoring of tissue gas tensions and pH in hemorrhagic shock. *Am. J. Surg.*, **126**, 249–254.

Niinikoski, J. (1980). Cellular and nutritional interaction in healing wounds. *Med. Biol.*, **58**, 303–309.

Niinikoski, J., Heughan, C. and Hunt, T.K. (1972). Oxygen tension in human wounds. *J. Surg. Res.*, **12**, 77–82.

Piasecki, C. (1985). First experimental results with the oxygen electrode as a local blood flow sensor in canine colon. *Br. J. Surg.*, **72**, 452–453.

Sheffield, P.J. (1988). Tissue oxygen measurements. In: Davis, J.C. and Hunt, T.K. (Eds), *Problem Wounds: The Role of Oxygen*, Elsevier, New York, pp. 17–51.

Sheridan, W.G., Lowndes, R.H. and Young, H. (1987). Tissue oxygen tension as a predictor of colonic anastomotic healing. *Dis. Colon Rectum*, **30**, 867–871.

Silver, I.A. (1969). The measurement of oxygen tension in healing tissue. In: Herzog, H. (Ed.), *Progress in Respiration Research. III.* Karger, Basel, pp. 124–135.

17

The Role of Oxygen in Wound Repair

JUHA NIINIKOSKI, FINN GOTTRUP[1] and THOMAS K. HUNT[2]

Department of Surgery, University of Turku, Finland, [1]Department of Surgical Gastroenterology K, Odense University Hospital, Denmark, and [2]Department of Surgery, University of California School of Medicine, San Francisco, California, USA

CELLULAR AND METABOLIC INTERACTIONS

A fundamental property of wounds aside from the disruption of connective tissues is the destruction of the nutritional supply to the tissue. The most fundamental property of *wound healing* together with restoration of connective tissue continuity is the restoration of its microcirculation. Neither can occur without the other. The characteristic structure of reparative tissue reflects the symbiosis between regenerating connective tissue and its neovasculature which must first support regeneration and later maintain scar. It follows that the signs of the local metabolic 'crisis' due to tissue injury should become signals for subsequent repair. It should also follow that repair will continue until the metabolic needs are met and tissue continuity is restored. The wound architecture is partly controlled by the energy needs of the wound cells. New wound capillaries are stimulated to migrate towards the hypoxic and acidotic area at the wound edge. Cells in the van of the advancing wound edge produce lactate, growth factors and chemotactic stimuli that diffuse back towards the developing microvasculature. The growth of new vessels needs stromal support. On the other hand, the fibroblasts which supply stromal support require nutrients to make collagen, fibronectin, and proteoglycans. Thus, in the wound milieu a delicate interaction exists between the inflammatory cells, new vessels and fibroblasts (Hunt and Halliday, 1980).

Reparative cells must necessarily migrate into the wound space. Migration usually occurs along concentration gradients, and steep concentration gradients are found in wounded and healing tissue. Extreme gradients of oxygen, carbon dioxide, pH, lactate, and glucose have been measured and others undoubtedly exist (Fig. 1). Measurements of oxygen tension gradients demonstrate that pO_2, which is of the order of 60–90 mmHg over the most

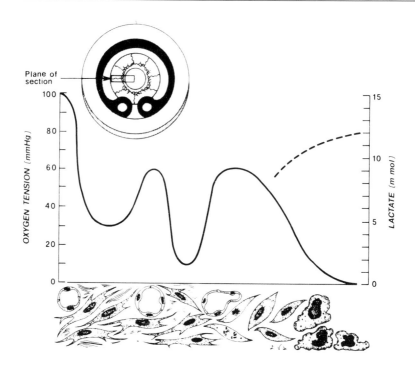

Figure 1. Side view of the advancing edge in a rabbit ear chamber. The oxygen tension profile is shown above. The pO$_2$ is high over the capillaries and nearly zero at the centre of the wound. Macrophages are the only cells which appear to tolerate such low oxygen tension. The central wound space remains hypoxic and acidotic despite approaching neovasculature. (Reproduce with permission, from Hunt and Van Winkle, 1979.)

distal capillary at the wound edge, decreases to near zero at the zone of macrophages and the central dead space (Silver, 1969; 1980; Niinikoski *et al.*, 1972). In the area of dividing fibroblasts, which is almost confined to the leading capillary zone, the pO$_2$ is in the region of 30–80 mmHg.

Almost no cell division can be found where the oxygen tension is consistently below 20 mmHg. According to Silver (1980), maximum synthetic and collagen cross-linking activity takes place in a zone in which the pO$_2$ is 20–60 mmHg and where the oxygen diffusion gradients are much less steep than those at the wound edge.

OXYGEN AND HEALING

The discovery that oxygen is a pivotal nutritional ingredient of healing has stressed the importance of efficient oxygen supply to the repair tissue. Studies

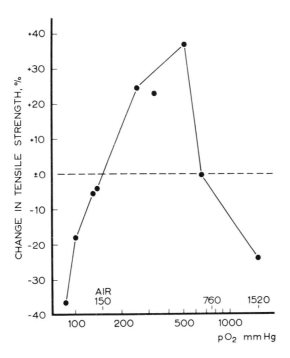

Figure 2. Effect of inspiratory oxygen tension on the tensile strength of healing skin incisions in rats 10 days after wound infliction. (Reproduced with permission, from Niinikoski, 1969.)

from several laboratories have shown that in many types of wounds increased oxygen tensions stimulate healing and, conversely, that reduction in available oxygen inhibits repair (Lundgren and Zederfeldt, 1969; Niinikoski, 1969; Silver, 1971; Stephens and Hunt, 1971; Hunt and Pai, 1972).

Niinikoski (1969) showed that the tensile strength of incisional wounds in rats increases as ambient oxygen concentrations increase from 18–70 volume per cent. When 70% oxygen was administered, the tensile strength was 35% above the control level in 10 day wounds (Fig. 2). Systemic hypoxia suppressed the healing rate, and the optimal conditions were passed when the oxygen treatment was extended to 100% oxygen at 1 ATA pressure or to hyperbaric oxygen at 2 ATA given intermittently in 2 hour periods twice daily. Parallel observations in subcutaneous cellulose sponge implants demonstrated that the favourable effect of oxygen resulted from (i) enhanced accumulation of collagen, (ii) slightly augmented cross-linking of collagen, and (iii) increased synthetic activity of wound cells, as indicated by a rise in their RNA/DNA ratio. These findings were confirmed by several investigators who showed that the oxygen effects apply to healing of ear chambers and wire mesh cylinders in rabbits and that not only strength and collagen deposition but also angiogenesis and epithelialization are enhanced. Recently, the effect has been demonstrated in wound models in man (T.K. Hunt, unpublished).

Collagen synthesis is crucially dependent on the availability of molecular oxygen. Oxygen is incorporated into the peptide chain to form hydroxyprolyl and hydroxylysyl residues. Hutton *et al.* (1967) found a close correlation between the rate of proline hydroxylation and oxygen concentration over the range of 0.51–14.9 volume per cent of oxygen by using a partially purified chick embryo hydroxylase. The K_m value for oxygen was 2.6 volume per cent, equalling a pO_2 of about 20 mmHg. These results were confirmed by Myllylä *et al.* (1977) and more recently challenged by De Jong and Kemp (1984) who suggest a higher figure. Partly because hydroxylation of proline is one of the terminal steps of collagen synthesis, its rate tends to limit the rate of collagen synthesis under most physiological conditions. If the nascent collagen peptides are not hydroxylated, they do not form the stable triple helix and are excreted from the cell as nonfunctional protein. The K_m (the concentration of a substrate which supports the rate of an enzyme at half its maximal value) in this case is roughly half the concentration which supports full velocity. This means that the synthesis of collagen will be limited by the oxygen tension in any fibroblast which exists in an extracellular environment in which pO_2 is less than about 50 mmHg. Theoretically, the effect will be most easily demonstrated in the range of 20–30 mmHg.

As shown in Fig. 3, the rate of collagen accumulation in healing wounds is a function of arterial pO_2 over a certain physiological range (Hunt and Pai, 1972). Niinikoski (1980) showed that the accumulation of collagen is definitely impaired at mean oxygen tension of approximately 20 mmHg. This value accords with observations made with ultramicro oxygen electrodes in rabbit ear chambers in which the minimal pO_2 in the area of newly formed collagen fibres is of the order of 20–30 mmHg (Silver, 1980). The ear chamber studies have also shown, however, that oxygen tensions in healing tissue are heterogeneous. Even in normal physiological circumstances, areas of oxygen tensions in the limiting range are found.

In primarily closed surgical incisions, the mean pO_2 usually exceeds the crucial level of 20 mmHg (Niinikoski, 1980). This raises a question: why does increased systemic oxygenation enhance the rate of gain in the tensile strength of primarily closed incision wounds even though they seeem to be above the critical pO_2 level for collagen accumulation? This could be a result of raising the oxygen tension in the areas in which it is critically low. Another explanation would be enhanced cross-linking of wound collagen under high oxygen environment. This is supported by Chvapil *et al.* (1968) who reported that cross-linking of collagen in chick embryo skin slices increased almost linearly when oxygen concentration in the incubation gas was elevated from

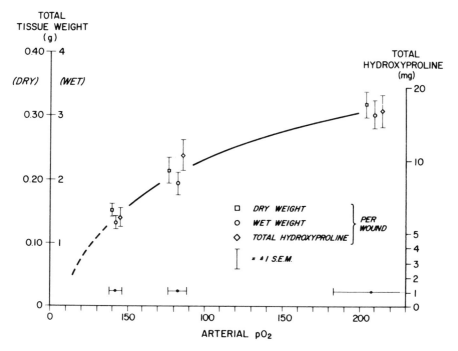

Figure 3.   Wound tissue and collagen as a function of arterial blood oxygen tension. (Reproduced with permission, from Hunt and Pai, 1972.)

20 to 95 volume per cent. Lysyl oxidase which catalyses some of the important covalent bonds which cross-link collagen peptides also uses molecular oxygen as a substrate. The critical or limiting range of oxygen tension is in the same range as in the case of prolyl hydroxylase.

THE CRITICAL ROLE OF LACTATE

The data pertaining to the influence of oxygen tensions on wound healing appear confusing and contradictory at first. On the one hand, hypoxia seems to be a stimulus to repair, and on the other hand, hyperoxia seems to stimulate components of repair. These 'contradictions' disappear when lactate concentrations are considered.

   Lactate levels in blood rarely rise over about 1 mmol/l in ordinary circumstances. In wounded tissue, they rise normally to the range of

5–15 mmol/l, and sometimes as high as 20 mmol/l. This would seem to be a consequence of hypoxia, but anaerobic glycolysis is only one contributor. Many wound cells, especially the macrophages (and possibly fibroblasts under the stimulus of interleukins) are aerobically glycolytic, i.e. produce and release lactate despite the presence of adequate oxygen to support aerobic intermediary metabolism.

At these high levels, lactate causes macrophages to produce and release an angiogenic substance (Jensen *et al.*, 1986). Furthermore, lactate leads to a reduction of synthesis of poly-ADP-ribose (from NAD^+) which ordinarily inhibits prolyl hydroxylase (Hussain *et al.*, 1989). Thus, the increased lactate enhances collagen synthesis and deposition as well as angiogenesis. When more oxygen is supplied, lactate levels in wounds fall only slightly, the lactate-mediated release of collagen synthesis is maintained, and a vital substrate which is in critically short supply is added. Furthermore, angiogenesis is enhanced (Knighton *et al.*, 1981) for unknown reasons.

These observations on lactate provide a theoretical basis in which the important role of energy deficit and supply can be seen as intercooperative with the role of inflammatory cells. The interaction may be even greater since there is some (unpublished) evidence that lactate also modulates the response of fibroblasts to growth factors.

SUPPLY OF NUTRITIONAL SUBSTANCES

In addition to oxygen, the supply of other nutritive substances is of vital importance for healing. Glycolysis, the pentose monophosphate shunt, the Krebs cycle, and oxidative phosphorylation all participate in the energy production of reparative tissues. Glucose is utilized abundantly through the pentose monophosphate shunt, especially in the early phases of healing when leukocytes predominate, and glycolysis dominates during the synthesis of collagen (Lampiaho and Kulonen, 1967).

The delivery of nutritional substances at the healing edge may be extremely precarious. It is possible that cells in the immediate vicinity of the most distal vessel consume glucose so extensively that the delivery to the most peripheral cells in the van of the advancing tissue is limited. It is attractive to speculate that this imbalance could be corrected by raising the mean capillary pO_2, which would suppress the glucose consumption of cells adjacent to capillaries by allowing metabolism to be more efficient (Niinikoski, 1977). Relatively more glucose would then become available for the most peripheral cells at the hypoxic zone. This could explain the observation that glucose utilization in healing wounds as a whole increases if added oxygen is available (Kivisaari *et al.*, 1975).

EFFECTS OF BLOOD VOLUME, ANAEMIA AND HAEMODILUTION ON WOUND HEALING

Changes in the circulating blood volume lead to dramatic alterations in the tissues. The new capillaries are extremely sensitive to conditions which affect tissue perfusion. On the other hand, fibroblasts in the resting stage appear to tolerate severe changes in environment, but those in a proliferative phase are extremely sensitive to such changes. Silver's (1973) findings in rabbit ear chamber wounds showed that the new vessels collapse upon withdrawal of blood from the animal. This happens before any fall in the systemic blood pressure is noted. In established shock, perfusion of the wound edge ceases almost entirely and the pO_2 declines to zero. After treatment of shock, perfusion of the area returns slowly and the tissue growth is suppressed for several days after the insult.

Overloading of circulation with fluid of low osmotic pressure results in oedema in the growing zone, which increases the diffusion distances between the capillaries. This in turn reduces the pO_2 on the surface of cells not immediately adjacent to capillaries and suppresses their mitotic rate (Silver, 1980). These findings confirmed and extended those of Heughan et al. (1972) who demonstrated a rather long-term decrease in the pO_2 of dead-space wounds after excessive saline infusions.

Several investigations have been carried out on the relation of anaemia to wound healing. Those methods of inducing anaemia which simultaneously result in hypovolaemia have suppressed collagen synthesis and healing, while methods of producing mild or moderate uncomplicated normovolaemic anaemia or haemodilution have not impaired repair or the delivery of oxygen to the wound. In tests of dead-space wounds in normal animals, a haematocrit of 30% with normal blood volume was found more suitable for repair than a haematocrit of 40% in terms of total collagen deposition in the wound space (Heughan et al., 1974). Looking at the tissue perfusion by means of local tissue pO_2 measurements, disturbance of wound microcirculation or oxygenation have not been observed during limited normovolaemic haemodilution, but a more homogeneous distribution of microcirculatory flow, most likely as a consequence of the reduced blood viscosity, has become apparent (Messmer, 1987; Hansen et al., 1989).

THE CRITICAL ROLE OF VASOMOTOR TONE

We have shown that although healing tissue depends on oxygen, it uses rather little, approximately 0.7 ml per 100 ml of arterial blood flow in a healing subcutaneous wound. We have also shown, however, that in order to be useful, the oxygen must be transported at a relatively high tension. This can be achieved only by a healthy heart and lungs and a rapid perfusion of the new vessels. In this case, the autonomic nervous system which supports the circulation to vital organs during stress is an enemy of repair because it tends to support central functions at the expense of perfusion of the connective tissues. Hypovolaemia is not the only means by which local circulation is diminished. Fear, pain, and especially cold are potent activators of vasoconstriction as are nicotine, and a number of cardio-active drugs such as adrenergic β-blockers. We have measured profound hypoxia in human test wounds during administration of excess epinephrine and local cooling. We have also measured hyperoxia during local warming. Drugs which might inhibit reflex vasoconstriction are, therefore, a target of great potential in the management of wound healing.

OXYGEN AND WOUND INFECTION

In surgery most problems and complications related to healing wounds are caused by infection. Wounds in poorly perfused tissues become infected far more often than wounds in well perfused tissues. An important mechanism by which white cells selectively kill bacteria uses oxygen. Wound hypoxia seems to suppress the function of this mechanism (Hunt, 1979). In hypoxic tissues even small increments in the available oxygen may result in relatively large increases in resistance to infection. For instance, experimental studies have demonstrated that the size of staphylococcal inoculum necessary to produce clinical infection is reduced when the wound pO_2 is decreased and is increased above normal when the wound pO_2 is increased (Hohn *et al.*, 1976). The mechanism for the oxygen effect on microbial killing by leukocytes is apparently similar to that of collagen synthesis. When leukocytes ingest bacteria, the so-called leukocyte primary oxygenase is activated. Molecules of oxygen are supplied with an additional electron to form superoxide. This is the initial step of an oxygen radical generation system in which the excess electron is passed on to various other molecules and eventually into bacterial cell walls. The K_m for oxygen of this enzyme is about 8 mmHg and the V_{max} is about 30–40 mmHg. This means that oxidative killing of bacteria is sensitive to pO_2 from 0 to about 30–40 mmHg. This mechanism accounts for about half of the leukocytes' capacity to kill staphylococci for instance.

SUMMARY

Whatever the signals which trigger the repair process, it is clear that the rate of healing is dependent on the local delivery of oxygen and other nutrients. New tissue growth is centred around blood vessels, which support new capillaries to supply the advancing cells. The endothelial buds grow towards areas of low oxygen tension, but they will not do so unless they have been preceded by macrophages. Macrophages probably act as director cells to provide chemotactic signals for endothelium to follow and to release stimulatory substances for fibroblast replication and 'activation'. The synthesis of collagen by fibroblasts seems to be crucially dependent on the availability of molecular oxygen as is the ability of endothelial cells to form new vessels. The main function of polymorphonuclear leukocytes in the wound is to resist infection. An important mechanism by which white cells selectively kill bacteria uses oxygen. Thus, any treatment that augments the local oxygen supply or helps to avoid hypoperfusion of the wound will tend to increase the rate of healing and decrease the susceptibility to infection.

REFERENCES

Chvapil, M., Hurych, J. and Ehrlichova, E. (1968). The influence of various oxygen tensions upon proline hydroxylation and the metabolism of collagenous and non-collagenous proteins in skin slices. *Z. Physiol. Chem.*, **349**, 211–217.

De Jong, L. and Kemp, A. (1984). Stoichiometry and kinetics of the prolyl 4-hydroxylase partial reaction. *Biochem. Biophys. Acta*, **787**, 105–111.

Hansen, E.S., Gellett, S., Kirkegärd, L., Hjortdahl, V. and Gottrup, F. (1989). Tissue oxygen tension in random pattern skin flaps during normovolemic hemodilution. *J. Surg. Res.*, **47**, 24–29.

Heughan, C., Niinikoski, J. and Hunt, T.K. (1972). Effects of excessive infusion of saline solution on tissue oxygen transport. *Surg. Gynecol. Obstet.*, **135**, 257–260.

Heughan, C., Grislis, G. and Hunt, T.K. (1974). The effect of anemia on wound healing. *Ann. Surg.*, **197**, 163–167.

Hohn, D.C., MacKay, R.D. and Hunt, T.K. (1976). The effect of oxygen tension on the microbicidal function of leukocytes in wounds and *in vitro*. *Surg. Forum.*, **27**, 18–20.

Hunt, T.K. (1979). Disorders of repair and their management. In: Hunt, T.K. and Dunphy, J.E. (Eds), *Fundamentals of Wound Management*, Appleton-Century-Crofts, New York, pp. 68–168.

Hunt, T.K. and Halliday, B. (1980). Inflammation in wounds: from 'laudable pus' to primary repair and beyond. In: Hunt, T.K. (Ed.), *Wound Healing and Wound Infection: Theory and Surgical Practice*, Appleton-Century-Crofts, New York, pp. 281–293.

Hunt, T.K. and Pai, M.P. (1972). The effect of varying ambient oxygen tensions on wound metabolism and collagen synthesis. *Surg. Gynecol. Obstet.*, **135**, 561–567.

Hunt, T.K. and Van Winkle, W., Jr (1979). Normal repair. In: Hunt, T.K. and Dunphy, J.E. (Eds), *Fundamentals of Wound Management*, Appleton-Century-Crofts, New York, pp. 2–67.

Hussain, M.Z., Ghani, Q.P. and Hunt, T.K. (1989). Inhibition of prolyl hydroxylase by poly (ADP-ribose) and phosphoribosyl-AMP. *J. Biol. Chem.*, **264**, 7850–7855.

Hutton, J.J., Tappel, A.L. and Udenfried, S. (1967). Cofactor and substrate requirements of collagen proline hydroxylase. *Arch. Biochem.*, **118**, 231–240.

Jensen, J.A., Hunt, T.K., Scheuenstuhl, H. and Banda, M.J. (1986). Effect of lactate, pyruvate, and pH on secretion of angiogenesis and mitogenesis factors by macrophages. *Lab. Invest.*, **54**, 574–578.

Kivisaari, J., Vihersaari, T., Renvall, S. and Niinikoski, J. (1975). Energy metabolism of experimental wounds at various oxygen environments. *Ann. Surg.*, **181**, 823–828.

Knighton, D.R., Silver, I.À. and Hunt, T.K. (1981). Regulation of wound-healing angiogenesis: Effect of oxygen gradients and inspired oxygen concentration. *Surgery*, **90**, 262–270.

Lampiaho, K. and Kulonen, E. (1967). Metabolic phases during the development of granulation tissue. *Biochem. J.*, **105**, 333–341.

Lundgren, C.E.J. and Zederfeldt, B. (1969). Influence of low oxygen pressure on wound healing. *Acta Chir. Scand.*, **135**, 555–558.

Messmer, K.F.W. (1987). Acceptable hematocrit levels in surgical patients. *World J. Surg.*, **11**, 41–46.

Myllylä, R., Tuderman, L. and Kivirikko, K.I. (1977). Mechanism of the prolyl hydroxylase reaction. 2. Kinetic analysis of the reaction sequence. *Eur. J. Biochem.*, **80**, 349–357.

Niinikoski, J. (1969). Effect of oxygen supply on wound healing and formation of experimental granulation tissue. *Acta Physiol. Scand.*, **334**, (Suppl.) 1–72.

Niinikoski, J. (1977). Oxygen and wound healing. *Clin. Plast. Surg.*, **4**, 361–374.

Niinikoski, J. (1980). The effect of blood and oxygen supply on the biochemistry of repair. In: Hunt, T.K. (ed.), *Wound Healing and Wound Infection: Theory and Surgical Practice*, Appleton-Century-Crofts, New York, pp. 56–71.

Niinikoski, J., Hunt, T.K. and Dunphy, J.E. (1972). Oxygen supply in healing tissue. *Am. J. Surg.*, **123**, 247–252.

Silver, J.A. (1969). The measurement of oxygen tension in healing tissue. *Progr. Resp. Res.*, **3**, 124–135.

Silver, J.A. (1971). Wound healing and cellular microenvironment. Final technical report. US Army Contract No. DAJA 37-70-2328.

Silver, J.A. (1973). Local and systemic factors which affect the proliferation of fibroblasts. In: Kulonen, E. and Pikkarainen, J. (Eds), *Biology of Fibroblast*, Academic Press, London, pp. 507–519.

Silver, J.A. (1980). The physiology of wound healing. In: Hunt, T.K. (Ed.), *Wound Healing and Wound Infection: Theory and Surgical Practice*, Appleton-Century-Crofts, New York, pp. 11–31.

Stephens, F.O. and Hunt, T.K. (1971). Effect of changes in inspired oxygen and carbon dioxide tensions on wound tensile strength. *Ann. Surg.* **173**, 515–519.

Clinical Wound Healing Research

Wound Healing
Edited by H. Janssen, R. Rooman and J.I.S. Robertson
© 1991 Wrightson Biomedical Publishing Ltd

18

A Strategy for Human Studies: Thoughts on Models

THOMAS K. HUNT, WILLIAM H. GOODSON III and HEINZ SCHEUENSTUHL

Department of Surgery, University of California, San Francisco, USA

This book brings together a group of investigators poised with new knowledge of the repair process which seems sufficient to make major contributions to patient care. However, it is clear that one of the major obstacles to exploitation of our collective knowledge is the lack of human models with which to test the potential clinical applications. This chapter addresses this problem first by assembling the information available on one of the two most useful human models of healing, and secondly, by proposing a strategy for research involving human subjects. This is the nuclear idea of a long-term, multi-institutional project which has been forming in our minds for several years.

The reasons for the paucity of research in human wound healing are not entirely clear. After all, man is easy to wound. Miniaturized methods can minimize the obvious problems of pain and disfigurement. There are many examples of important clinical research in other fields which have involved far greater danger and discomfort. The problem is rather that in approaching human research, there must be a high degree of expectation of results. A new standard of creative criticism must be adopted and the investigator must ask again what, in fact, will be learned and how important will be the new knowledge? Unfortunately, our profession as a whole is reasonably satisfied with the status quo with regard to healing. In the estimation of many, nothing very important is likely to be learned from clinical research on wound healing. Secondly, those of us who would do the investigations are seriously divided about what can be learned. There is a somewhat mysterious feeling that human models have little relevance to human wounds. We suspect that this stems from the current preoccupation with chronic wounds and a precipitous rush for what we call 'bottom line' kinds of answers.

It is commonly accepted that there are many important benefits of deliberately influencing human repair, and it is as well to remember that our profession was several times before so satisfied with the status quo that it greeted the work of Paré, Lister, and Semmelweis with considerable hostility. In order to make progress we must now reach agreement on the kind of information that might arise from the human models. Disagreements lie mainly in the perceived shortcomings of the various models. In our opinion, every wound model has shortcomings: all models fall short of global realization of repair. We might thus be able to agree on a strategy to attack clinical problems by accepting that: (i) components of repair can be measured individually, and (ii) surrogate models can be devised in human patients. This requires some explanation.

COMPONENTS OF REPAIR

Strategically it is important to think in terms of components of repair. Wounds are heterogeneous. There are big ones, small ones, open ones, closed ones, deep ones, shallow ones, bony ones, etc. Some wounds heal mainly by epithelialization, some mainly by contraction, some by simple collagenous union, and some by replacement of large amounts of new tissue, etc. One can distinguish six different processes which contribute. They often overlap, and each can be subdivided, but the basic elements appear to be inflammation, cell replication, epithelialization, angiogenesis, matrix deposition, and contraction. The interaction of these elements makes it difficult for one wound to serve as an example of another. The wound site may limit one or another of the components. For examples, contraction is limited in an area of tight skin. However, models which emphasize each of these components have been devised. Several components are remarkably susceptible to direct measurement. If we can isolate each component, we have the opportunity to optimize it within the capacity of the patient population.

By thinking in terms of components, we may be able to give up the criticism that any given model fails to take into consideration one or more components of repair. Instead, we can seek out deliberately models which emphasize or clearly isolate only one or another component. The rationale is that by subdivision, we can eliminate unnecessary complexity and will then be free to compare only results which are indeed comparable.

SURROGATE WOUNDS

The second part of the strategy is to devise surrogate wound models within the framework of measuring components. The old statement, 'to make a difference, there must be a difference' has held back clinical wound healing research for many years. Translated into terms of clinical research, it says that unless actual wound complications are used as the end point of a clinical study, the result cannot be accepted as valid or significant. If this limited perspective continues to hold, each and every improvement in management of human wound healing will await studies of hundreds, and perhaps thousands, of patients with all the frustration and complexity which that necessitates.

On the other hand, surrogate wounds can be used. They can relate an objective measure of one or more components of repair to actual clinical events. This will require a few large studies. Thereafter, however, with the principles proved, perturbations such as growth factors or nutrition, for instance, can be linked to the objective data obtained from the surrogate. Clinical significance can be judged by the degree to which the components are changed with respect to their individual significance in the exploratory studies. For instance, we have just shown (unpublished) that wound infections are extremely rare when (surrogate) wound oxygen tension can be raised over about 70 torr by breathing oxygen. With that information, we can now study various interventional strategies in terms of wound pO_2 and infer an effect on infection. Whatever strategy raises wound pO_2 to that level is likely to increase resistance to infection. Strategies which are effective at this level can be tested with confidence against the actual incidence of infection later. Since surgical technique is not a factor in the surrogate, we will be able to distinguish, at last, between patient- and surgeon-derived variables. No doubt, there are hazards in this approach, but without it, there can only be limited hope for clinical research.

We have explored the avenue of surrogate wounds far enough to be certain that it is already an effective strategy. Viljanto (1990) is even further advanced than we in his study of literally thousands of wounds with his 'cellstick' method. This method, a tiny cellulose sponge implant, measures mainly aspects of the inflammatory response and to some extent cell replication. With it, he has been able to distinguish patient populations which are at risk for wound complications.

In summary, until recently human wound healing has been measurable only in overt complications – infections, dehiscences, excessive scar, hernia, fistula, malunions, etc. These can be disastrous problems, and if human healing must forever be measured in such terms and in no other way, many patients will be hurt in the process. We hypothesize, without fear of contradiction, that in the background of all these complications there are measurable deviations from normal repair which can be defined in terms of the components of healing.

A MODEL

In order to test this hypothesis, we developed a simple, soft tissue wound model for use in patients along the lines of previous 'space' models. We tried for a model which could isolate inflammation, cell replication, and matrix deposition and synthesis which would have the following specifications: (a) a small sampler which can be inserted and removed painlessly; (b) fabrication from a substance which excites a minimal foreign body reaction; (c) a pore size small enough to allow easy removal but large enough not to limit ingrowth of tissue; (d) a lumen which will accept the addition of such test substances as growth factors; (e) a gas-permeable matrix so that the thin wound sections which grow into it can be studied in tissue culture; (f) softness to allow microscopic sectioning; and (g) reproducibility in operation. The 90 and 120 μm spacing extruded, porous polytetrafluorethylene (teflon) tube (ePTFE) with a 1 mm outside diameter met these standards (Goodson and Hunt, 1982).

In experimental surgery, similar devices have been the most revealing of all wound models. Nevertheless, questions of the significance of the implant arise. In response to these questions, we offer the following: is the implant excessively inflammatory? Some investigators have found giant cells around ePTFE when collagen and growth factors were placed in the lumen (Sprengel et al., 1987), but when it is implanted empty, they are rare (Clark et al., 1974). Other, older implants such as polyvinyl chloride sponge incite more inflammation than ePTFE which ranks with dimethylsiloxan (Silastic) as the most noninflammatory plastic implantables known. Giant cells have been seen outside the mesh of PTFE implants, but not in the interstices. 'Normal' human subcutaneous wounds contain giant cells. We examined five specimens of breast biopsy sites excised 7–14 days after biopsy as a part of mastectomy. All contained a few giant cells. Some giant cells are a part of the 'real world' of wound healing.

Does the implant limit ingrowth of healing tissue? Several investigators have found the 90 μm spacing acceptable to reparative ingrowth. It has produced reproducible results in clinical and animal tests. The local conditions in this method are probably closer to those of 'normal' wounds, if there is such a thing, than any such model to date because the PTFE, in contrast to other implantable sampling methods, allows gases to diffuse unhindered and fluids to flow through its pores. Gas diffusion constants of polyvinyl, for instance, are far smaller than PTFE. Oxygen tensions in the central space of the tube span the same range as the same wound of implantation without the PTFE. PTFE has a nonwettable, nonadherent surface. This is as it should be since the 'normal' wound space also contains no adherent foreign body. In 'normal' wound spaces reparative tissue advances in a fibrin matrix. This matrix easily fills the PTFE pores and nutrient cells migrate in it. Studies have shown that 30 μm pore size limits ingrowth of tissue, but 120 μm pore size allows little if any more ingrowth than 90 μm material (Goodson, 1987). This is roughly three times the pore size of vascular grafts. Our choice of 90 or 120 μm size represents a compromize between easy penetration by new tissue and a fabric strong enough not to break in patients during insertion and removal.

In effect, PTFE is almost 'invisble' in tissue. In one sense this is a problem. Without added inflammatory stimulus, the yield of new tissue in the PTFE tube is rather low (as it was in polyvinyl sponges until Pernokas and Dunphy learned to implant them wetted with distilled water). Fortunately, sensitive analytical methods make this relatively low yield easily measurable. Use of water irrigation in this method, too, seems to increase yield and reduce variability.

Is the matrix which is deposited in ePTFE typical of wounds? The extracellular matrix retrieved from grafts in both fetal and adult implants contains hydroxyproline and hydroxylysine. Cyanogen bromide fragments from it are consistent with collagen and its common subtypes (Siegert et al., 1989). Upon ex vivo culture of tubes removed after periods in situ we find replicating cells which take up radiothymidine, convert radiolabelled proline to hydroxyproline, and incorporate radioactive sulphate to glycosaminogly-cans (Rabkin et al., 1986). Extraction of collagen by acetic acid, with subsequent salt precipitation and dialysis, leaves a weighable residue which chromatographs as collagen and contains the radioactive hydroxyproline which is converted during incubation of the tube with radioproline (unpublished). Examination with transmission electron microscopy shows fibres with cross-striations typical of collagen, and typical fibroblasts, macrophages, and endothelial cells. Examination with histochemical stains shows typical collagen staining with Mallory's trichrome (microscopic observations are not yet published).

In summary, the ePTFE model can measure pertinent components of repair and can quantify changes in wound healing without the need to incur and count complications. In particular, the model measures inflammation, fibroplasia, and matrix synthesis. It does not measure epithelialization at all. We cannot say how well it reflects contraction. There are no current assays of angiogenesis in wounds, but the model would seem to be amenable to proposed methods of doing so.

Can the ePTFE assay actually make distinctions with regard to repair? It already has an excellent record. Using this technique, the following have been demonstrated:

1. Cells replicate and deposit matrix faster in fetuses than in newborn infants, while newborns mobilize these components faster than their mothers (Adzick et al., 1986).
2. Animals mobilize component cells faster, begin collagen deposition sooner and begin resolution sooner than does man (Goodson and Hunt, 1982; Rabkin et al., 1986).
3. Collagen deposition is normal in well-controlled diabetic patients compared with normal controls (Goodson and Hunt, 1984).

4. Obese, hyperglycaemic mice deposit collagen less rapidly than do their lean littermates (Goodson and Hunt, 1986). In the latter instance, less collagen in the PTFE correlated with a quantitatively similar defect in contraction.
5. Hypoxic and poorly perfused patients deposit collagen poorly (Jonsson *et al.*, 1986).
6. Placement of alginate in the centre of PTFE tubes increases collagen deposition (unpublished). DNA and thymidine assays show clearly that the increment is due to increased inflammation, that is, DNA content was markedly elevated while thymidine incorporation was only moderately elevated.

The model can also discriminate between classes of patients who are at risk for poor healing and complications of repair. As noted above, hypoxic and poorly perfused patients deposit collagen poorly. To examine the implications of this, we have shown that:

1. Collagen in the subcutaneous PTFE model in pigs and rats correlates closely with tensile strength of other, primarily closed skin wounds in the same animals (unpublished).
2. Although poor collagen deposition by no means characterizes all patients with recurrent hernias, we have found it in three of the 10 patients with recurrent hernias that we have studied. So far, dehiscences have been confined to a group with very poor collagen deposition.
3. Patients with anaemia uncomplicated by cardiac or respiratory disease heal normally (Jensen *et al.*, 1986).
4. Smokers deposit collagen less rapidly then do nonsmokers (Goodson and Hunt, 1984).
5. A brief pre-operative illness (which inhibits nutrition) suppresses collagen deposition (Goodson *et al.*, 1987).
6. Malnourished patients deposit less collagen than normals and are significantly improved by intravenous nutrition (Haydock and Hill, 1987).
7. Uraemic patients deposit collagen more slowly than normal controls (Goodson *et al.*, 1982).
8. Recently, and without precedent, Barbul *et al.* (1990) have shown that normal men deposit collagen considerably faster if they take oral arginine.

No other dead-space wound model has ever been subjected to such close scrutiny with regard to clinical relevance. In summary, the data from the use of the PTFE model recapitulate surgical expectations and experience.

Method

Two ePTFE tubes, each 5–6 cm long, are implanted, at operation or under local anaesthesia, in the upper arm. The PTFE is threaded on to a long cutting needle and placed in the subcutaneous space into one stab wound and out another 5–6 cm proximal. A small segment is left protruding from the entrance or exit wound. A 5–0 nylon stitch is placed to fix the tube in position. In contrast to an earlier method, we now place single lengths instead of doubled lengths.

The tube is harvested at 7 or 10 days by pulling it out after clipping the nylon stitch. All dry tube is discarded. If the specimen is destined only for measuring collagen deposition it is frozen immediately. At a later time the tube is placed in a 60°C oven overnight, then hydrolysed in 6 N HCl for 18 hours at 188°C. The hydrochloric acid is then removed and the dissolved specimen is analysed for total hydroxyproline by the method of Grant (1967). If culture data is desired each pair of catheters is removed and trimmed to precisely equal lengths. They are separated and each is placed in 1 ml Dulbecco's modified Eagle's medium containing penicillin, streptomycin, neomycin, 50 μg/ml ascorbic acid and 10% vol/vol NuSerum (Collaborative Research Products). One tube is radiolabelled with 1 μCi/ml 1-(2, 3, 4, 5) $-^{14}$C-proline (Amersham) for three hours at 37°C. The other is placed in the same culture material without the uniformly labelled proline, but instead with 10 μCi/ml methyl-^{3}H-thymidine (New England Nuclear) for 3 hours at 37°C. Each sample is washed five-fold with 0.2% cetylpyridinium chloride solution in deionized water, after which all are placed in a 60°C oven overnight. One ml of 6 N HCl is added to the proline-labelled group, and the samples hydrolysed at 110°C for 18 hours. After hydrolysis the supernates are dried at 60°C over a bed of sodium carbonate. After 36 hours the dry samples are rehydrated with 1.2 ml of deionized water. Four hundred μl are used to assay total hydroxyproline, 100 μl to determine counts per minute of ^{14}C, and 400 μl for the manual hydroxyproline method of Kivirikko et al. (1967) using Peterkofsky et al.'s (1962) method of separating radiolabelled proline from hydroxyproline.

For this assay the samples are brought up to 0.5 ml. One-half gram solid KCl, 0.25 ml 10% β-alanine and 0.5 ml potassium borate buffer (pH 8) are added and the samples mixed. One-half ml of 10% chloramine-T is added for 25 min. One ml of 1 M $Na_2S_2O_3$ then stops the reaction. Two extractions with 3.0 ml of toluene remove free proline. The samples are then heated to 100°C for 30 min. After cooling, two additional extractions with 3 ml toluene are done. Counts per minute are determined on the residual aqueous sample and the pooled toluene extract. One ml of Erlich's reagent is added to 2 ml of the toluene extract and colour allowed to develop for 20 min at room temperature. The optical density at 560 nm is determined against a reagent blank and total hydroxyproline against a standard curve run in parallel. The total hydroxyproline measured correlates ±5% with that obtained by the method of Grant (1967).

One ml of 4°C 0.5 N $HClO_4$ is added to the ^{3}H-thymidine-labelled group, and it is allowed to sit at 4°C for 50 min to remove free thymidine and to precipitate DNA. The supernate is decanted, and counts per minute and uronic acid content determined (Bitter and Huir, 1962). One millilitre of 0.5 N $HClO_4$ is added to the sample, which is heated to 100°C for 15–20 mins. After cooling, 100 µl is used for counting, 200 µl to determine total uronic acid content, and 500 µl to determine total DNA by the method of Burton (1956).

Interpretation

We interpret the results of the hydroxyproline assay as a measure of the collagen which has been deposited in the PTFE fabric. We are pursuing more detailed proof. We interpret DNA as the sum of inflammation and cell replication. We interpret thymidine uptake as an indirect measure of the number of replicating cells, i.e. fibroblasts and endothelial cells (Rabkin *et al.*, 1986). Thus, we can estimate (a) the degree of inflammation, (b) the degree of fibroplasia, (c) the degree of matrix deposition, and (d) therefore, the 'efficiency' of fibroblast mechanisms.

Virtues of the PTFE model are (i) the model is acceptable to human subjects; only one patient in 300 has asked for premature removal of the tube; (ii) the method is versatile; we can measure total DNA, total sulphate uptake, collagen synthesis, collagen synthetic capacity, and thymidine uptake under standardized culture conditions; (iii) questions of pathophysiology can be examined (Rabkin *et al.*, 1986).

PRIOR STUDIES

This model is singularly useful and important because there have been few objective, quantitative studies of human wound healing. The first was done by DuNouy who, in 1937, reported studies done in the First World War in which he measured the open area of cutaneous wounds over a period of time and successfully delineated the roles of age and intercurrent infection in the rate of healing of such acute open wounds. Sandbloom *et al.* (1953) studied tensile strengths of incised and sutured wounds on the human forearm. This also detected the effect of age. Paries *et al.* (1967) used a cast model to study the effect of zinc on open wounds. Viljanto (1990) has done yeoman's work with another sponge dead-space model in which he has made the kind of correlations we feel are possible using mainly the inflammatory component of repair as a guide. This model should also be used in multi-institutional studies. Many surgeons have counted infections and dehiscences, of course, and data are beginning to appear on the effects of growth factors on open wounds (Brown *et al.*, 1989). Most of these studies examine only 'bottom lines' and not components. This is attractive from the perspective of industry, but it almost eliminates the possibility of mechanistic explanations emerging. In the short time that it has been available, the ePTFE model has more than doubled our knowledge of human wound healing, and it has been used by a number of investigators.

WHAT CAN AND CANNOT BE GAINED?

The idea I have outlined is a beginning. This kind of approach will not answer all questions nor will it meet all expectations. For instance, in order to obtain a full view of human repair, the remaining components of healing will need study as well. Models of epithelialization have been developed. Contraction models should not be difficult. Angiogenesis remains unmeasured in man. Clearly, with this strategy, multiple models will be necessary; and if the best advantage is to be taken, some agreements on their use should be made among us. Since circulation dominates repair, there will be regional differences. Wounds on extremities will be particularly sensitive to vasomotor changes. The ideal site(s) remain(s) to be determined. The Viljanto (1990) model should either be included or the 'cellstick' and the ePTFE models should be fused.

These ideas reflect our general assumption, based on considerable data, that wound healing in surgical patients is commonly impaired. Large, multi-institutional studies with models of human wound components can show why and how much it is hindered and whether the problem is malnutrition, malperfusion, inflammatory suppression, etc. Specific nutritional remedies can be sought as Barbul *et al.* (1990) are doing. The effects of cold, vasoactive drugs, immune suppressants, length of surgery, etc., can be tested with minimal reference to actual complications. The next projects in our laboratory will deal with growth hormone, insulin-like growth factor I, and vasoactive pharmaceuticals.

Lastly, models such as these will have limited immediate relevance to the current preoccupation with chronic wounds, but they will continue to be immediately relevant to the major postoperative/post-traumatic problems which so often lead to disability and even death. In view of the features of the ePTFE model, however, a number of answers about the effects of 'growth factors' and other mediators of repair in humans should result.

We propose that one of the first functions of the American and European Wound Healing Societies should be a working group to plan and initiate multicentre, international studies on human repair.

ACKNOWLEDGEMENTS

This work was supported by grant No. GM27345-10 from the General Medical Sciences Institute of the National Institutes of Health.

REFERENCES

Adzick, N.S., Harrison, M.R., Glick, P.L., Beckstead, J.H., Villa, R.L., Scheuenstuhl, H. and Goodson, W.H. (1986). Comparison of fetal, newborn, and adult wound healing by histologic, enzyme-histochemical, and hydroxyproline determinations. *J. Pediatr. Surg.*, **20**, 315–319.

Barbul, A., Lazarou, S., Efron, E.T., Wasserkrug, H.L. and Efron, G. (1990). Arginine enhances wound healing in humans. *Surgery*, **108**, 331–337..

Bitter, T. and Muir, M. (1962). A modified uronic acid carbazole reaction. *Anal. Biochem.*, **4**, 330–334.

Brown, G.L., Nanney, L.B., Griffen, J., Cramer, A.B., Yancey, J.M., Curtsinger III, L.J., Holtzin, L., Schultz, G.S., Jurkiewicz, M.J. and Lynch, J.B. (1989). Enhancement of wound healing by topical treatment with epidermal growth factor. *N. Engl. J. Med.*, **321**, 76–79.

Burton, K. (1956). Study of conditions and mechanisms of diphenylamine reaction for colorimetric estimation of deoxynucleic acid. *Biochem. J.*, **62**, 315–323.

Clark, R.E., Boyd, J.C. and Moran, J.C. (1974). New principles governing the reactivity of prosthetic materials. *J. Surg. Res.* **16**, 510–522.

DuNuoy, P.L. (1937). *Biochemical Time*, MacMillan Co, New York.

Goodson, W.H. (1987). Application of expanded polytetrafluoroethylene (ePTFE) tubing to the study of human wound healing. *J. Biomaterial Applications*, **2**, 101–117.

Goodson, W.H. and Hunt, T.K. (1982). Development of a new miniature method for the study of wound healing in human subjects. *J. Surg. Res.*, **33**, 394–401.

Goodson, W.H. and Hunt, T.K. (1984). Wound healing in well-controlled diabetic men. *Surg. Forum*, **35**, 614–616.

Goodson, W.H. and Hunt, T.K. (1986). Wound collagen accumulation in obese, hyperglycemic mice. *Diabetes*, **35**, 491–495.

Goodson, W.H., Lindenfeld, S.M., Omachi, R. and Hunt, T.K. (1982). Chronic uremia does cause poor healing. *Surg. Forum*, **33**, 54–56.

Goodson, W.H., Lopez-Sarmiento, A., Jensen, J.A., West, J., Granja-Mena, L. and Chavez-Estrella, J. (1987). The influence of a brief preoperative illness on postoperative healing. *Ann. Surg.*, **205**, 250–255.

Grant, R.A. (1967). Estimation of hydroxyproline by the Auto Analyser. *J. Clin. Pathol.*, **17**, 685–686.

Haydock, D.A. and Hill, G.L.; Improved wound healing responses in surgical patients receiving intravenous nutrition. *Br. J. Surg.*, **74**, 320–323.

Jensen, J.A., Goodson, W.H., Vasconez, L. and Hunt, T.K. (1986). Wound healing in anemia: A case report. *West. J. Med.*, **144**, 465–467.

Jonsson, K., Jensen, J.A., Goodson, W.H. and Hunt, T.K. (1986). Wound healing in subcutaneous tissue of surgical patients in relation to oxygen availability. *Surg. Forum*, **37**, 86–88.

Kivirikko, K.I., Laitinen, O. and Prockop, D.J. (1967). Modification of a specific assay for hydroxyproline in urine. *Anal. Biochem.*, **19**, 249–255.

Pories, W.J., Henzel, J.H., Rab, C.G. and Strain, W.H. (1967). Acceleration of wound healing in man with zinc sulfate by mouth. *Lancet*, **i**, 121–124.

Peterkofsky, B. and Prockop, K.J. (1962). A method for the simultaneous measurement of the radioactivity of proline-C-14 and hydroxyproline-C-14 in biological materials. *Anal. Biochem.*, **4**, 400–406.

Rabkin, J., Hunt, T.K., Von Smitten, K. and Goodson, W.H. (1986). Wound healing measurement by radioisotope incubation of tissue samples in PTFE tubes. *Surg. Forum*, **37**, 592–594.

Siegert, J.W., Burd, D.A.R., McCarthy, J.G., Weinzweig, J. and Ehrlich, H.P. (1989). Fetal wound healing: Biochemical studies of scarless healing. *Plast. Reconstruct. Surg.*, **85**, 495–502.

Sandbloom, P.H., Peterson, P. and Maren, A. (1953). Determination of the tensile strength of the healing wound as a clinical test. *Acta Chir. Scand.*, **105**, 252–257.

Sprugel, K.H., McPherson, J.M., Clowes, A.W. and Ross, R. (1987). Effects of growth factors *in vivo*. I: Cell growth into porous subcutaneous chambers. *Am. J. Pathol.*, **129**, 601–613.

Viljanto, J.A. (1990). Assessment of wound healing speed in man. In: Barbul, A., Caldwell, M., Eaglstein, W., Hunt, T.K., Marshall, D., Pines, E. and Skover, G. (Eds), *Clinical and Experimental Approaches to Dermal and Epidermal Repair: Normal and Chronic Wounds*, Allan R. Liss, New York, 1990.

Wound Healing
Edited by H. Janssen, R. Rooman and J.I.S. Robertson
© 1991 Wrightson Biomedical Publishing Ltd

19

A Scientific Approach to Wound Measurement: The Role of Stereophotogrammetry

M.S. WALSH and A.W. GOODE

Surgical Unit, The London Hospital, Whitechapel, London, UK

INTRODUCTION

Chronic open wounds such as leg ulcers and pressure sores are a common problem. An estimated 0.4 million people suffer with leg ulcers in Britain (Callam *et al.*, 1985) and a recent survey at the London Hospital revealed that 3% of the inpatients developed pressure sores prior to or during their admission (B. Thompson, 1989, personal communication). The treatment of these wounds consumes large quantities of resources in terms of personnel, time and money, often with poor results (Monk and Sarkany, 1982). A major difficulty is deciding the most appropriate treatment from the large number that are available: Bulstrode encountered more than 100 treatments for leg ulcers (Bulstrode, 1986). This diversity is partly explained by the lack of a universally available, objective means of measuring wounds and their healing rates.

The problem of wound measurement is a recurring theme when considering wound healing studies. These difficulties lead to inaccurate and often subjective comparisons between treatments. As a consequence it is difficult to interpret the findings of healing studies. Superficially the most appropriate method of circumventing these problems would be to utilize the time to complete healing as the main criterion in wound healing studies. This approach however has several drawbacks. First, the time to complete healing of a wound is often difficult to define. This can be appreciated if we consider the small area of crusting persisting on many wounds after the majority has re-epithelialized. Secondly, the time and expense of performing large statistically powerful studies would be prohibitive since many wounds, even in ideal circumstances, take weeks and often months to heal. Finally, this method excludes assessments of the intermediate stages of healing, therefore making patterns of healing and predictive models difficult to develop and the assessment of treatments aimed at the intermediate stages of healing would be inadequate.

There is, therefore, an urgent need to develop an accurate and precise method of measuring wounds and healing rates. Such a system would enable objective comparisons of treatments, delineation of healing patterns and potentially the development of predictive wound healing models and mapping of tissues within a wound.

The requirements of a wound measurement technique need to be defined before proceeding with the development of a new system. The requirements for such a system are that it is:

(a) accurate, so that true values for wound measurements are obtained;
(b) precise, that is repeated measurements give a reproducible result;
(c) non-invasive, so that there is no direct contact with the wound, therefore avoiding pain, contamination and disruption of delicate healing tissues;
(d) quick and easy to use since many medical staff are not technically trained; further, patients with chronic wounds are often old and frail and do not tolerate long complicated techniques easily;
(e) able to measure volume, area and circumference to allow complete healing models to be developed and to assess the volume in relation to healing rates;
(f) able to produce results at the time of measurement to facilitate clinical decision making; and
(g) adaptable to storage and retrieval of the results from a database.

Examples of wound measuring techniques currently available include plain photography plus planimetry (Myers and Cherry, 1970), direct tracing plus planimetry (Burnand et al., 1980), ultrasound digitization (Coleridge Smith and Scurr, 1989), and measurement of diameters (Baker and Haig, 1981). None of these techniques fulfils the criteria above. Main drawbacks include poor accuracy and precision, direct contact with the wound, and inability to measure all three dimensions with one technique. For clinical trials and healing research the problems of inaccuracy and imprecision are paramount and arise from the two-dimensional approach of these techniques to a three-dimensional problem.

STEREOPHOTOGRAMMETRY

In the Surgical Unit at The London Hospital there is an interest in the metabolism of the tissues within a wound and the correlation of this with healing patterns and rates. These types of correlation are beyond the measurement techniques currently available. To overcome the problems of wound measurement it was decided to investigate a number of possibilities and the technique which appeared to have the most potential to fulfil the measurement criteria was stereophotogrammetry. This is a technique developed in the middle of the last century for map making and surveying. With developments in photography, measuring devices and computers, the applications of stereophotogrammetry have expanded to include engineering, architecture, archaeology and medicine, particularly when three-dimensional measurement is required. Examples of medical uses include measurements for facial and breast reconstructions, retinal measurement, dentistry and assessment of prosthetic hip loosening.

Stereophotogrammetry requires two photographs of an object to be taken from different perspectives. A three-dimensional image of that object can then be formed by the brain, providing the image of each photograph is passed to its respective eye. Measurements can then be made either directly from this image or by calculation using the co-ordinates of equivalent positions on the two photographs. These techniques are described as metric and analytical, respectively. Normal vision is stereoscopic because the brain creates a three-dimensional image of the viewed object by comparing the small differences between the images on each retina due to the different perspective of each eye. In stereophotogrammetry the creation of the perspective difference is performed one step removed from the eye by the use of two cameras. The advantage of this is that differences of perspective are fixed in time by the photographs so allowing measurements to be made.

Pilot study of stereophotogrammetry

A pilot study comparing conventional wound measuring techniques and stereophotogrammetry was performed at The London Hospital. The conventional techniques studied were direct tracing with planimetry and plain photography with planimetry. Stereophotogrammetry was performed using an adapted stereocamera and a reflex metrograph. The metrograph was manually operated and measurements were taken directly from the three-dimensional image and recorded by digital encoders which passed the information to a computer. Calculations of wound circumferences, area and volume were performed by the computer using a mathematical model.

Each measuring technique was assessed for accuracy and precision. Accuracy was assessed by making repeated measurements of model ulcers of known size and by then calculating the percentage error of the mean. Precision was assessed by making repeated measurements of real leg ulcers and then calculating the coefficients of variations. A sample of the results is given in Tables 1 and 2. In addition stereophotogrammetry was able to provide measurements of wound volume (Table 3).

Table 1.   Accuracy errors of pilot study (%
error of the mean of known areas).

Area (mm^2)	Tracing	Photography	SPG[a]
10.0	60.0	43.0	0.9
50	29.0	23.0	0.6
140	16.5	10.7	0.6
405	10.0	16.0	0.9
790	5.8	8.6	0.8
1200	0.3	3.9	1.1
2050	3.7	1.6	1.0
3260	5.8	4.0	1.0
4540	4.0	3.2	0.7
6380	2.9	5.1	0.7
9840	0.4	10.0	0.7
14 110	2.3	8.5	0.6
Mean	11.7	21.0	0.8

[a]SPG = stereophotogrammetry.

Table 2.   Precision errors of pilot study (95%
confidence intervals as a % of mean).

Area (mm^2)	Tracing	Photography	SPG[a]
8	48.0	45.7	5.5
12	37.8	19.6	3.8
15	60.3	47.7	4.3
16	19.0	9.1	5.9
16	64.6	66.0	1.9
82	29.0	21.6	2.7
92	57.0	36.0	3.1
114	17.0	11.0	2.0
125	21.6	14.1	1.8
134	23.4	15.9	2.6
Mean	37.8	28.6	3.36

[a] SPG = stereophotogrammetry.

The accuracy and precision of stereophotogrammetry was far superior to
that of the conventional techniques. The improvement in accuracy and
precision with stereophotogrammetry was sustained across the range of
wound sizes. This is of particular relevance in wound healing studies since
healing rates decrease as wounds become smaller and errors at this stage
would greatly affect trial results. Furthermore, stereophotogrammetry was
able to produce reliable volume data and the accurate measurements
obtained were used to produce a wound healing model for chronic leg ulcers.

Table 3. Volume measurement by
stereophotogrammetry (accuracy and precision errors).

Volume (mm^3)	Accuracy error (%)	Precision error (%)
10	5.4	1.0
58	5.2	2.1
210	4.9	2.5
823	4.7	2.5
3860	5.8	1.2
10 220	5.7	1.3
26 150	5.6	1.1
60 440	5.6	2.2
103 400	5.8	2.4
223 300	4.8	1.9
413 280	5.2	1.3
649 000	4.7	1.3
Mean	5.2	1.3

This model enabled a prediction of the time to complete healing to be made after 3 weeks of treatment.

The results for stereophotogrammetry in the pilot study were very promising. However, its use as a research and clinical tool was severely limited by the problems with the equipment, i.e. by the inconvenience of the camera and the reflex metrograph. It was decided that the system needed to be redesigned if stereophotogrammetry was to achieve its potential in wound healing problems. The aim was to design a system that would not only provide the accuracy and precision required but would also fulfil the other criteria for a clinical measuring system. The equipment used and the results obtained in the pilot study are more fully discussed in the papers describing this work (Bulstrode *et al.*, 1986; 1987).

DEVELOPMENT OF THE NEW SYSTEM

The camera

The new camera (Fig. 1) is a hand held metric stereo-camera with the two camera boxes on an aluminium base plate. The cameras are built from commercially available lenses, shutters and film carriages. This gives variable apertures and shutter speeds making extra lighting unnecessary. Film loading, winding on and shutter release are conventional and mechanical in operation.

The camera has several additional features to facilitate clinical use. For range finding and to ensure the object is in the field of view an intersecting light system, operated by a switch on one of the camera handles, has been

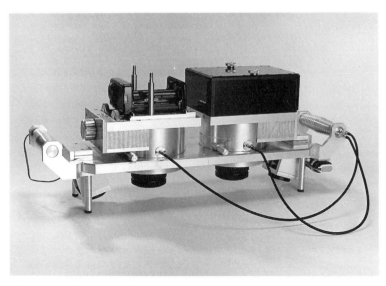

Figure 1. Redesigned stereocamera with one camera box removed.

designed. To minimize errors due to film distortion the films are flattened against a glass plate by a spring mechanism. During winding on the pressure on the film is relieved by a cam system incorporated into the wind on mechanism, which lifts the film carriage. The glass plates have crosses etched into them which act as the fiducial marks (reference points). This eliminates the need for an external frame carrying these marks, as was the case with the original camera. The design of the camera means that it is light, portable and easy to use. From the patient's point of view taking the photographs is quick and non-invasive.

The analytical measuring system

The measurement system has been changed from metric to analytical, which involves calculation of the three-dimensional co-ordinates from equivalent positions on the two photographs. This has enabled the development of an automated system, controlled by a computer. As a consequence the effort, time and errors of measurement have been reduced.

The system is based on a stereomicroscope. The two photographs are mounted on an orthogonal slide system and each image is passed to its respective eyepiece of the microscope by a system of mirrors (Fig. 2). By orientating the two photographs correctly a three-dimensional image floating in space is seen through the microscope (Fig. 2). There are four slides which allow four movements in two planes (Fig. 3). Each slide is moved by a motor

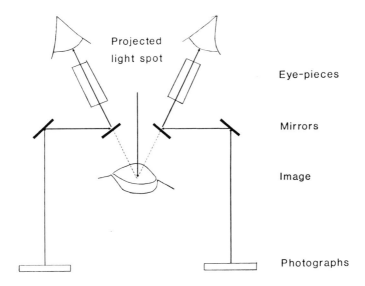

Figure 2.   Image formation in the stereomicroscope.

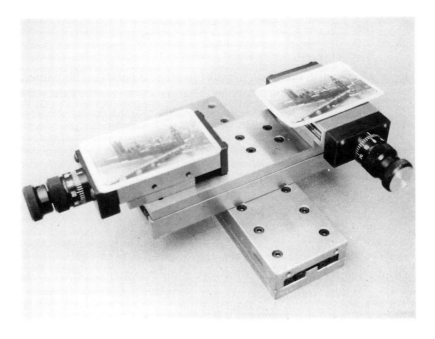

Figure 3.   Mock up of the orthogonal slide system to show the orientation of the slides and photographs.

which is controlled by the computer. The computer is an IBM compatible personal computer together with a customized interface for the microscope. The movements of each slide are recorded by digital encoders which pass the information to the computer for calculation in the rewritten mathematical model.

For calculation of wound size, a three-dimensional image needs to be described in a digital form. This is achieved by selecting points on the image of the wound and the surrounding skin visually and calculating their co-ordinates. To select points, a fixed light spot is projected on to the image. The image is moved in three dimensions around the light spot, while viewing it through the microscope, by use of a track ball and unidirectional wheel. The track ball gives movements in the x–y plane and the unidirectional wheel gives movements in the z direction. When a selected point of the image is correctly positioned on the light spot a foot switch is pressed to record its co-ordinates.

The slide system (Fig. 3) is arranged so that gross movements of the two photographs in the x and y directions are carried out together; these movements will be called X_s and Y_s. Each photograph is mounted on a separate slide, to allow differential movements. These movements called dx and dy also occur in the x and y directions, respectively. The mathematical explanation for this arrangement and its consequences are beyond the scope of this chapter. However an intuitive understanding can be obtained if we consider a cube and two two-dimensional representations of it from different perspectives (Fig. 4).

The translation from A to B on the cube is described in three dimensions by the movements X, Y, Z. However, in the two-dimensional representations the same translation of A to B is described by the movements X_1, Y_1 and X_2, Y_2, respectively. From this we can deduce two main points:

(a) the two sets of two-dimensional translations and co-ordinates uniquely describe equivalent translations and co-ordinates in three dimensions, providing the orientation of the two-dimensional representations to each other is known. The calculations to provide the three-dimensional co-ordinates from two-dimensional data involve over 30 steps and are performed by the computer. The orientation of the photographs in the system is fixed by the positions of the fiducial crosses etched into the glass plates of the cameras and subsequently reproduced on the photographs.

(b) The translations X_1, Y_1 and X_2, Y_2 are not necessarily equal in value due to the differences in perspective and therefore a means of differential movement is required. This is provided by the dx and dy slides on which the photographs are mounted.

The complete system works in the following manner (Fig 5); prior to taking co-ordinates from the three-dimensional image the two fiducial crosses are

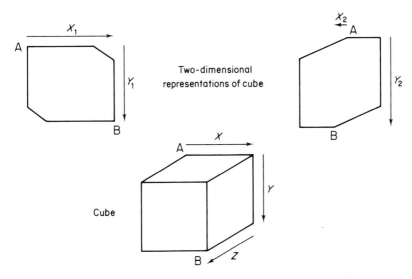

Figure 4. Translation of two-dimensional co-ordinates to three-dimensional co-ordinates (see text for explanation).

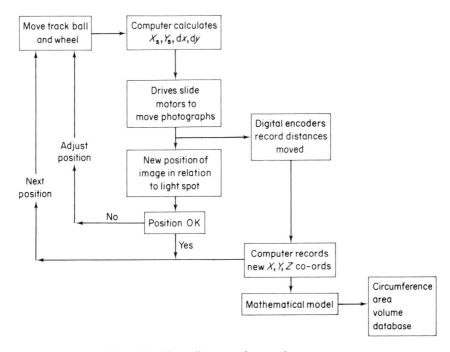

Figure 5. Flow diagram of operating system.

identified and the image is moved so that each is placed in turn under the light spot and their position is recorded by pressing the foot switch. The computer now has a frame of reference which fixes the orientation of the photographs, since the relative positions of the fiducial crosses is the same for every pair of photographs and the computer is programmed with this information. The computer is now informed of the intention to move to the first chosen point on the three-dimensional image by the operator moving the track ball and unidirectional wheel. The computer interface calculates what this represents in terms of the two-dimensional movements required for each photograph. The computer than instructs the slide motors to move their respective slides the appropriate amounts of X_s, Y_s, dx and dy.

If the chosen point has been correctly positioned under the light spot the computer is informed by pressing the foot switch, otherwise the position is adjusted by further movements of the track ball and unidirectional wheel. After the foot switch has been pressed the computer records the three-dimensional co-ordinates of the chosen point and the image can be moved to the next position. The speed of the computer means that the time between adjusting the controls and seeing the image move is minimal.

The scanning of the wound images is carried out in a series of parallel sweeps (Fig. 6). The first point chosen is on the epithelial margin at the side of the wound. The first sweep is then performed a short distance along the wound in the x direction. The wound image is then moved only in the y and z directions to produce a longitudinal sweep across the wound.

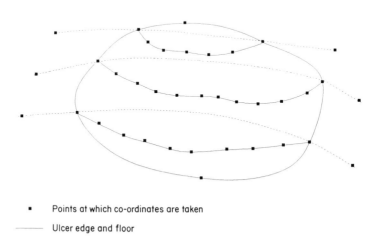

•   Points at which co-ordinates are taken

———   Ulcer edge and floor

....   Third order curves

Figure 6. Diagramme of wound scanning and third order curves (spacing between scans and points exaggerated).

The first point in a sweep is taken on the normal skin surrounding the wound. The second point is taken on the epithelial margin and then a series of points in the wound base, the far epithelial margin and finally the normal skin on the far side of the wound. When a sweep has been completed the wound is moved along a short distance in the x direction and the process is repeated until the complete wound has been scanned.

Points can be selected from any part of the wound and at any distance apart because the mathematical model which calculates the wound parameters utilizes random points. Therefore it is possible to take into account any prominent features and changes of contours within a wound.

The computer

The computer performs three separate functions in the measurement system:

Image movements

The interface box is programmed to interpret instructions from the track ball, unidirectional wheel and the foot switch. The instructions from the three-dimensional controls are converted into two-dimensional movements of the photographs, from which the co-ordinates of the new position on the image are known. The co-ordinates are then passed to the programme for the mathematical model.

Calculation

The calculations of wound circumference, area and volume from the co-ordinates are performed by a mathematical model which recreates the wound from the co-ordinates. The programme has been rewritten to incorporate an improved model, therefore reducing errors. The circumference of the wound is calculated by summing the distances between all the points selected on the epithelial margin. The distances between adjacent points are calculated by trigonometry. The area of the wound is calculated by triangulation incorporating all the points recorded on the wound margin and base.

The volume of a wound is calculated by first recreating the skin surface which would have been present if the wound had not occurred. This is achieved using the points on normal skin and the two points on the epithelial margin of each sweep, to give the third order curve which uniquely fits these four points (Fig. 6). In this way the skin surface corresponding to each sweep is recreated. The sweeps are made longitudinally to reduce the errors of forming the third order curves. This is because on the leg and at many of the pressure points of the body the degree of curvature longitudinally is less than the transverse curvature. A series of perpendiculars is produced from each point in the wound floor to its respective third order curve. Using these perpendiculars, whose heights are calculated by subtraction, a series of irregular prisms with parallel sides is formed across the wound. The volume of each prism is calculated and then they are summed together to give the wound volume.

As mentioned previously, one of the advantages of the improved mathematical models is that they utilize randomly spaced points and sweeps thus making it possible to describe fully the features of a wound. The final accuracy obtained in measuring a particular wound increases with the number of points and sweeps made. However a balance is reached because of the limits of the equipment, the visual acuity of the operator and the time taken to process an image. Expected errors in accuracy and precision for this equipment with a processing time of about 15 min are in the order of 1%.

Data storage

The computer is able to produce a graphical impression of each wound on the screen and this can be compared directly with previous scans of the same wound. This opens up the possibilities for wound mapping and comparison of healing in different areas of a wound. The wound measurements, patient details and wound graphics are stored in a database. This will allow comparisons to be made between wounds, treatments and different aetiologies. The amount of data should allow good healing models to be developed.

PROJECTED USES OF STEREOPHOTOGRAMMETRY IN WOUND HEALING

The expected errors have been discussed above; however work is presently under way to define the accuracy and precision in a similar manner to that in the pilot study. The system now fulfils all the criteria for a clinical measurement technique except that results are not immediately available because of the need for film processing. This should not be a problem in research. The major benefits are clinical acceptability for both patient and doctor, the ease of processing the images, the small errors and the possibilities for studying factors affecting healing rates.

The equipment is presently being used to study the efficiency of topical ketanserin for wound healing. We are also intending to use it for mapping wounds and for correlating the healing in specific areas of a wound with measures of the local metabolism such as tissue oxygen and laser Doppler flowmetry.

Stereophotogrammetry has the potential to become the 'gold standard' in wound measurement and we are currently undertaking joint projects with two dermatology departments to compare our system with conventional wound measurement techniques in animal wound healing models. To standardize wound healing research several centres could each own a stereocamera and the stereophotographs could be analysed at a central point. This would reduce both the expense of setting up the system and variation due to operator error. This type of collaboration in wound measurement could act as the focus for directing further wound healing research.

ACKNOWLEDGEMENTS

We would like to thank Mr C.K.J. Bulstrode who performed the majority of the work in the pilot study and Dr P.J. Scott of Reflex Measurements, Butleigh, Somerset for his considerable assistance with both stereophotographic systems.

REFERENCES

Bulstrode, C.J.K. (1986). *The use of stereophotogrammetry to measure the rate of healing in skin defects.* M. Chir. Thesis, University of Oxford.

Bulstrode, C.J.K., Goode, A.W. and Scott, P.J. (1986). Stereophotogrammetry for measuring rates of cutaneous healing: a comparison with conventional techniques. *Clin. Sci.*, **71**, 437–443.

Bulstrode, C.J.K., Goode, A.W. and Scott, P.J. (1987). Measurement of prediction of progress in delayed wound healing. *J. R. Soc. Med.*, **80**, 210–212.

Baker, P.G. and Haig, G. (1981). Metronidazole in the treatment of chronic pressure sores and ulcers. *Practitioner*, **25**, 569–573.

Burnand, K.G., Clemenson, G., Morland, M., Jarrett, P.E.M. and Browse, N.L. (1980). Venous lipodermatosclerosis: treatment by fibrinolytic enhancement and elastic compression. *Br. Med. J.*, **280**, 7–11.

Callam, M.J., Ruckley, C.V., Harper, D.R. and Dale, J.J. (1985). Chronic ulceration of the leg: extent of the problem and provision of care. *Br. Med. J.*, **290**, 1855–1856.

Coleridge Smith, P.D. and Scurr, J.H. (1989). Direct method of measuring venous ulcers. *Br. J. Surg.*, **76**, 689.

Monk, B.E. and Sarkany, I. (1982). Outcome of treatment of venous stasis ulcers. *Clin. Exp. Dermatol.*, **7**, 397–400.

Myers, M.B. and Cherry, G. (1970). Zinc and the healing of chronic ulcers. *Am. J. Surg.*, **120**, 77–81.

Summary

20

Aspects of Wound Healing: A Summary

J.I.S. ROBERTSON

Department of Medicine, Prince of Wales Hospital, Chinese University of Hong Kong, and Janssen Research Foundation, Beerse, Belgium

At the symposium on which this book is based, we were regaled with a wealth of information derived from superb biochemical, pharmacological and tissue culture studies. However, it appeared to me, and this impression was confirmed by several speakers, that the science of wound healing is not yet sufficiently advanced for a simple, unified and coherent set of concepts to be formulated. Most of the reasons are evident, cogent, and, albeit with some difficulty, in my opinion surmountable.

An initial problem concerns the definition and classification of wounds. The various speakers did not neglect this problem, and both Lapière and Hunt, in particular, addressed it most carefully. Nevertheless, difficulties remain. Whatever definition is adopted of a wound, the latter involves, necessarily, a disturbance of normal physiology. Therefore inevitably, difficulties of standardization are imposed.

Lapière opened the meeting by formulating some illuminating concepts, thus:

'Healing can be regarded as a homeostatic function, led by mesenchymal cells, and facilitating the subsequent organization of epithelial cells.'

'Healing involves local processes of chemotaxis, differentiation and multiplication, regulated by both chemical and physical mediators: these processes are analogous to growth, development, and ageing.'

'Ulcers can be regarded simply as disorders of healing.'

I found these ideas perceptive and helpful, although the notions became less lucid, and hence less valuable to me, during the debates in the course of the meeting. However, despite these reservations, some simple and largely uncontroversial requirements were propounded as described below.

The nature of a wound, and of its healing, should take account of the species, organ, and tissues involved. This precept was unfortunately not always followed at the meeting. For example, of concern to me was that analogies were drawn between hepatic cirrhosis and the healing of cutaneous wounds. Insufficient attention was paid to some probably very important structural and biochemical differences between healing in liver and skin.

Wounds can and should be classified according to whether a foreign body is present, whether they are infected and, if so, with what organisms; and whether they lie in situations hypoxic, ischaemic, neuropathic or diabetic. The age of the host and of the wound can both be important.

The nature and relevance of laboratory models require to be carefully defined and evaluated. Thus Davidson and others debated entertainingly on some important differences between various available artificial sponges in experimental models.

These several ideas were argued and developed during the course of the meeting. A simple time-table of skin healing was proposed, and not greatly disputed, thus:

(1) removal of debris and bacteria,
(2) extracellular matrix formation,
(3) vascular restoration with accompanying cellular changes.

We heard some superb accounts of the identification and chemical characterization of various growth-promoting factors, of growth inhibitors, and of processes which regulate the interactive balance between them. I trust that it will in no way detract from these excellent papers to state that in several respects I found that the biochemistry was running ahead of quantification. In making this point I am of course heavily influenced by my own background which has, for the past 20 years or so, been concerned with traditional endocrinology. This approach involves the measurement of the concentrations of the relevant hormone in the circulation, and then relating those concentrations to acute and long-term effects on target organs. This quantitative approach not rarely demonstrates that matters are not always as they may seem on superficial scrutiny. For example, the peptide vasopressin is an extremely powerful pressor agent, and it might therefore be supposed that it could have important effects in controlling arterial pressure in normal physiology, and also possibly be involved in the pathogenesis of some forms of hypertension. However, quantitative evaluation has not supported such predictions; only in some extreme circumstances, such as haemorrhagic hypotension, does sufficient vasopressin circulate peripherally to support arterial pressure.

Such precise, quantitative biochemistry was largely wanting at the symposium, a problem which was specifically recognized by several speakers, including Nicolas and Klagsbrun. It is of course very much more difficult to perform hormonal dose-response studies in tissues such as the skin, and especially in wounded skin, than it is in the circulation.

Another classic approach of traditional endocrinology, of studying syndromes resulting from excess or deficiency of a particular hormone, has been largely denied to those interested in wound healing, or has at most had limited exploitation. Lapière and Davidson agreed that genetic deletion of a substance critical for wound healing would often prove lethal early in life, thus restricting the opportunities for study. However, genetically-determined diminution, rather than absence of, a particular factor does offer valuable possibilities. Moreover, the likelihood that partial deficiency of wound healing substances might occur with ageing is not only likely, but also susceptible to scrutiny. So far this aspect has been little pursued.

These various critical comments are in no sense intended as denigration. We heard of some most elegant biochemical studies, but we do need to learn more of the clinical relevance of the findings.

We also heard from Klagsbrun and Woodley amongst others of uncertainties regarding the purity of some of the growth factors under study in wound healing. Such concerns are understandably inevitable. Similarly the reports of Barbul and of Nicolas indicated that occasionally mixtures, for example of cytokines, are involved in their experiments. Krieg dealt with cytokine regulation of collagen metabolism during wound healing.

Sank emphasized the important role of platelet-derived growth factor (PDGF) in angiogenesis and wound healing. We also heard descriptions of some exciting studies on inactive precursor peptides of PDGF. This work raises the intriguing possibility of activation of PDGF at specific sites in response to particular requirements.

Banda described the role of tissue inhibitors of metalloproteinases in regulating angiogenesis.

Seuwen presented a detailed and intricate account of studies on cultured hamster lung fibroblasts. He had detected receptors on the cell surface linked to two separate signalling pathways initiating cell growth. He had identified the groups of external growth factors acting on the surface receptors, and had elucidated the intracellular pathways responding to these receptors. The two pathways could work independently or synergistically according to need. This work offers the promise of a very exact means of studying the effects of drugs on healing. This report was supplemented and extended by the paper of Ryan.

There were other areas where quantification was less difficult. Niinikoski, Gottrup and Hunt had all made major inroads into the measurement of, and the establishment of the clinical relevance of, local tissue oxygen tension.

Tooke and Fagrell similarly delineated the importance of variations in the capillary circulation.

I did find it surprizing that on what might be supposed to be fairly straightforward histological issues, there remained considerable controversy. Thus it was stated that the fibroblast is 'elusive and difficult to define', a notion that was explicitly supported by Gabbiani. However, it was also held that the fibroblast 'is the primary cell at the heart of the healing process'. There seemed herein, at least to me, to exist a minor paradox, which I should prefer was resolved.

Further histological controversy was initiated by experimental and therapeutic studies in which cultured keratinocytes had been used to heal defects in skin. It was implied, without being stated explicitly, that the cultured keratinocytes produced more, and more effective, growth factors than did those of the host. It was further said that regeneration of dermis took up to 5 years to be completed. This latter statement was questioned by Rudolph and by Hunt, who wondered whether it was 'real dermis'. However, others said that they had caressed some of these patients and that they felt wonderful (to them). It remained unclear whether thermoregulation or touch sensation was fully restored. The presence of elastin, which it was specifically claimed might take up to 5 years to reappear after grafting, was asserted by Davidson but denied by Woodley. This particular controversy can presumably be fairly readily resolved.

I shall close with the reminiscence that there is a famous apocryphal case of wound healing dating from the tenth century, which has geographical associations with the venue of this symposium. According to Richard Wagner, Parsifal, a therapeutic innocent, spends a great deal of time (in legend many years; in the opera several hours) seeking the Roman spear with which Christ on the cross was stabbed. Eventually he succeeds, and, in combat with Klingsor, recovers the spear. The spear has remarkable curative properties, unfortunately for our present purposes not characterized in detail. When applied by Parsifal to the chronic wound of Amfortas, healing takes place within minutes. The local association is that Parsifal's second son, Lohengrin, married Elsa of Brabant in Antwerp cathedral, only a few kilometres from Corsendonk. The marriage was unfortunately not a success, but that is another story. It would however, be valuable if we knew more about the spear.

Index

209